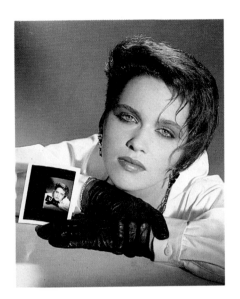

THE HAMLYN
BASIC GUIDE TO

Make-up

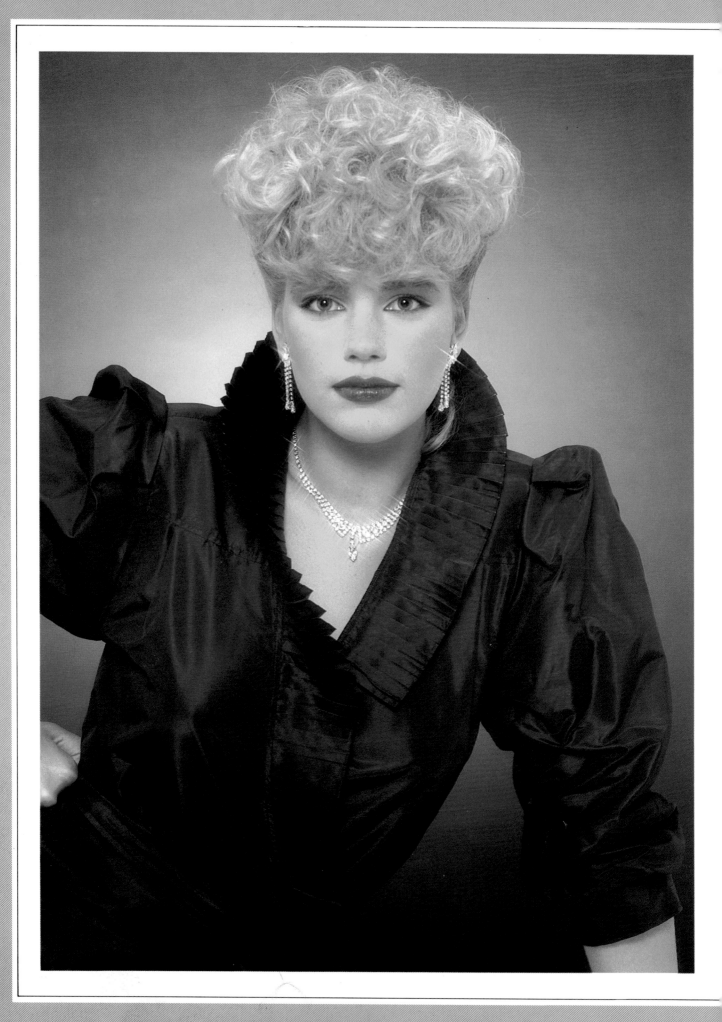

THE HAMLYN
BASIC GUIDE TO

Make-up

Jan Kettle

TREASURE PRESS

First published in Great Britain in 1986 by
The Hamlyn Publishing Group Ltd

This edition published in 1989 by
Treasure Press
Michelin House
81 Fulham Road
London SW3 6RB

ISBN 1 85051 403 8

Printed in Hong Kong

Half title page: Once you've learnt a few basic make-up rules, it's easy
enough to play up or down your look of the day to enhance your
mood. This dramatic look is courtesy of Alan International.

Title page: Some stunning evening looks may seem as if they've taken
hours to create, but that shouldn't be so. Ten minutes should be all
you need to transform an everyday look into something like this.
Picture courtesy of Hair & Beauty magazine.

Contents

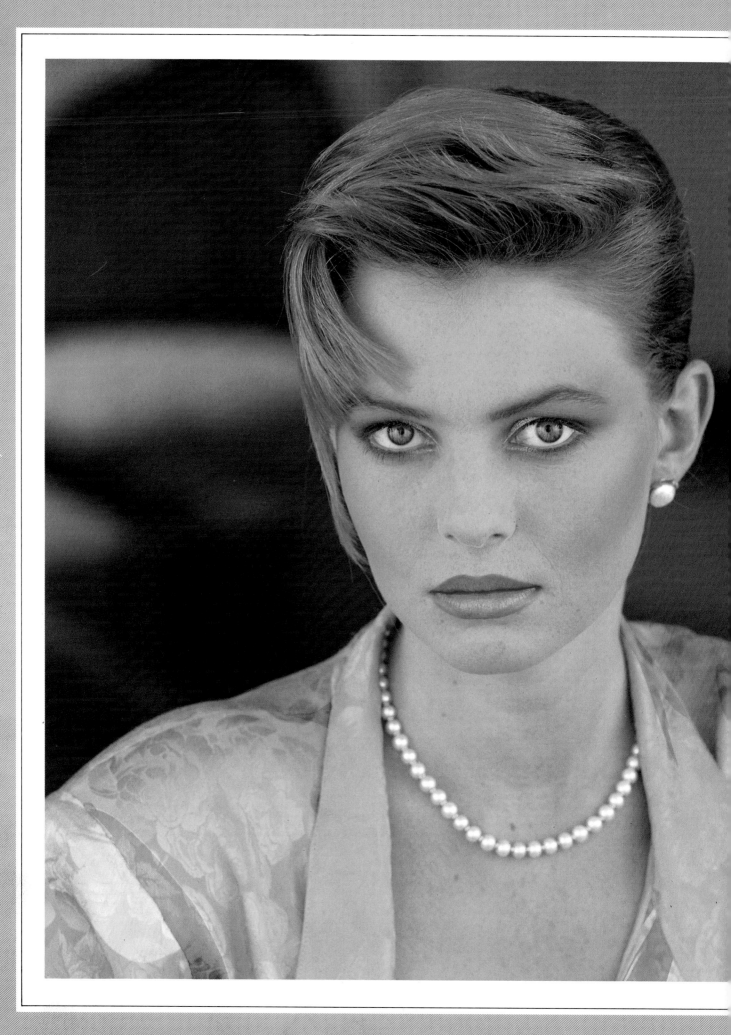

Introduction

Along with our hair and the clothes that we wear, make-up is one of the easiest and most effective ways of expressing to the world how we feel about ourselves. It reflects our character, our personality, our strengths and weaknesses and even our moods. Yet so often I see women who have misused and abused cosmetic products, simply because they don't understand them or how to use them. Glossy magazines offer a wealth of ideas on application, and keep us up to date on colours and trends in make-up, but they mostly tend to assume that we all know how to expertly apply these products.

As a make-up addict and someone who has made many mistakes herself, I started this book with a desire to explain the very basics of make-up: what it is, how to select the correct type for your skin, how to know what colours suit, and how to apply it. I asked myself all the questions I would like to have had answered when, as a teenager, I first started using make-up, but instead had to find out about the hard way. More than anything else I hope I can impress upon you that, although make-up can be used to enhance good features and disguise the not-so-good ones, it should be used as an interpretation of the way you feel about yourself and as a reflection of your personality, never as a mask.

Leave camouflage make-up to actors and actresses; the sort we use is for the real world. It should tell the people we meet in the course of a day something about ourselves, not hide or deceive. So be brutal. Sweep your hair off your face and take a good long look in the mirror in natural daylight. Ask yourself which part or parts of your face you would really like to highlight. Be positive about yourself rather than negative. If your eyes look wonderful the chances are that no one will ever notice that broad nose or double chin. Once the analysis is over, read on, and let your face do the talking.

Let your make-up reflect your mood and the way you feel about yourself. It can mirror your personality but never let it dominate. Photograph courtesy of Max Factor from their Colorfast 1980s Colour Cosmetic Range.

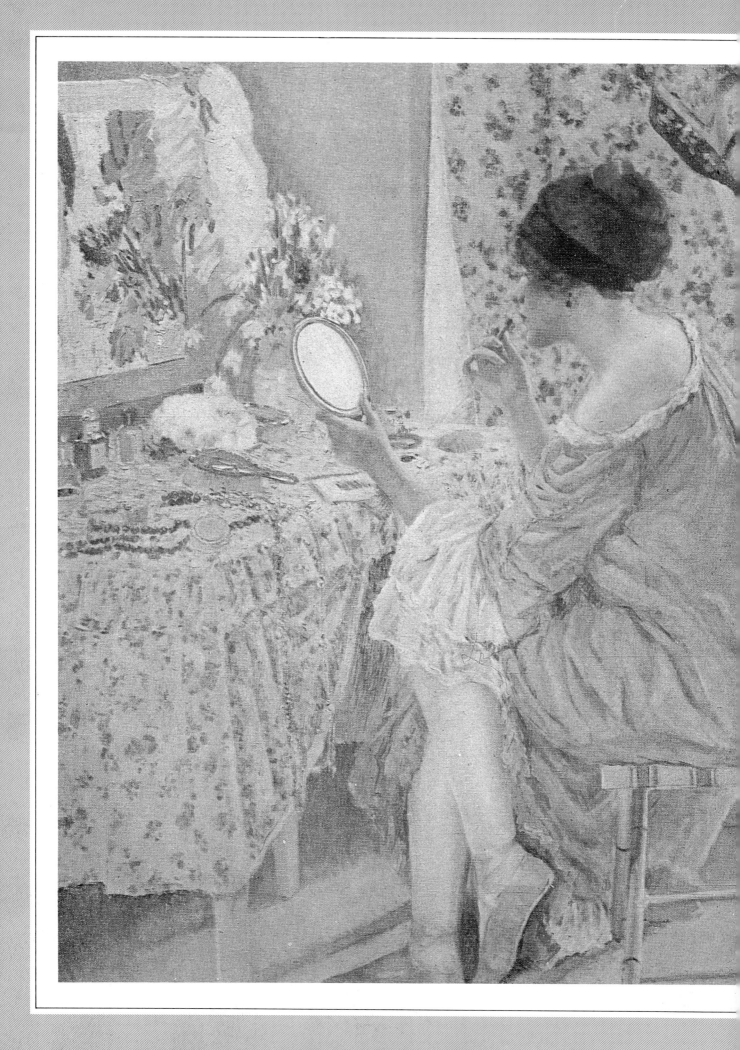

The history of make-up

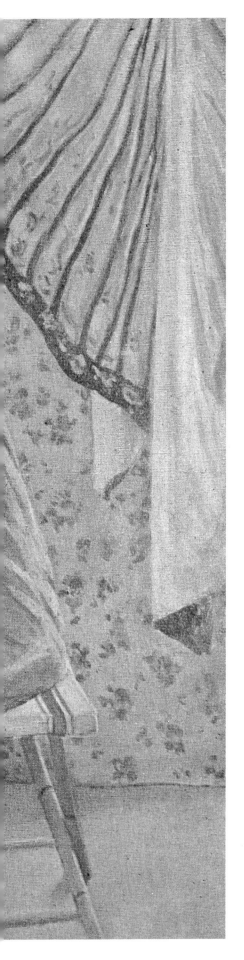

The majority of women spend on average 15 to 20 minutes a day making-up. 'Putting on' a face is as much a ritual. to most of us as dressing and brushing our teeth, and the way our face looks is our signature. It completes our total image and makes a statement about the way we feel about ourselves. Make-up enhances our personality and, because it has obviously taken time to put on, reflects the kind of discipline necessary for complete good grooming. There is also a great deal of artistry involved in making-up. It is the one aspect of a woman's appearance which gives her a chance to be creative, and when you look at how long make-up has been a ritual, it's no wonder this playground for creativity is so popular.

Cleansing and face painting played a great part in the early Middle Eastern and Mediterranean civilizations; we know from paintings and manuscripts that all the early cultures liked to accentuate their eyes and make them the most prominent facial feature. Egyptian eye make-up mainly consisted of malachite, a green ore of copper, and galena, a dark grey ore of lead, which were prepared by grinding them in a stone slab and placing the compound in a container. Cheeks and

Face painting has been popular since early times, but people in Britain were slow to catch on and cosmetics weren't really evident until the Middle Ages. Picture courtesy of the Mary Evans Picture Library.

lips were dyed with a mixture of red ochre combined with fat or oil. Ancient Greek courtesans used lavish make-up as a mark of their trade, and would add rouge to faces whitened with lead powder and eyes outlined with kohl.

People in Britain remained puritan for longer than most countries, and frowned heavily upon face painting, considering pale and natural to be pretty and perfect. Medieval women took this idea of perfection so far that they would even pluck all the hair from their eyebrows, temples and necks.

Cosmetics first came into use in Britain with the accession of Queen Elizabeth, whose pale complexion became the prototype for beauty. White powder was soon the essential cosmetic treatment, and was made either from alabaster or starch with added perfume, or white lead (the toxic effect of which had the most drastic results). Red ochre was used for rouge, and lips were painted with a pencil made from ground alabaster or plaster of Paris, powdered down and mixed into a paste with colouring ingredient. This was rolled into a crayon shape and then allowed to dry and solidify in the sun. These not very subtle Elizabethan faces were then preserved by covering the whole face with a thin glaze of egg-white, providing, should a lady venture out, a mask which protected against the sun, the bane of the fashionable white complexion.

In ensuing years, despite changes in fashion, make-up remained

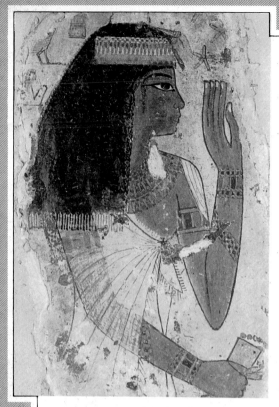

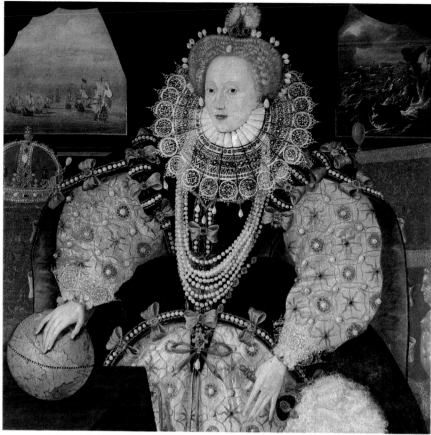

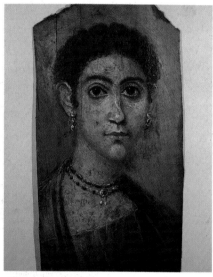

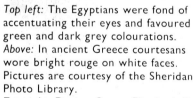

Top left: The Egyptians were fond of accentuating their eyes and favoured green and dark grey colourations.
Above: In ancient Greece courtesans wore bright rouge on white faces. Pictures are courtesy of the Sheridan Photo Library.
Top right: During Queen Elizabeth I's reign pale complexions were popular. White lead powder was the essential beauty aid despite its disastrous effects on health. Photograph courtesy of the Bridgeman Art Library.
By the 18th century (right) white powder was still widely used despite causing numerous ailments. Picture courtesy of the Mansell Collection.
Opposite: Marlene Dietrich epitomizes the style of the early 20th century: bright, cupid-bow lips and thin eyebrows. Picture courtesy of the Kobal Collection.

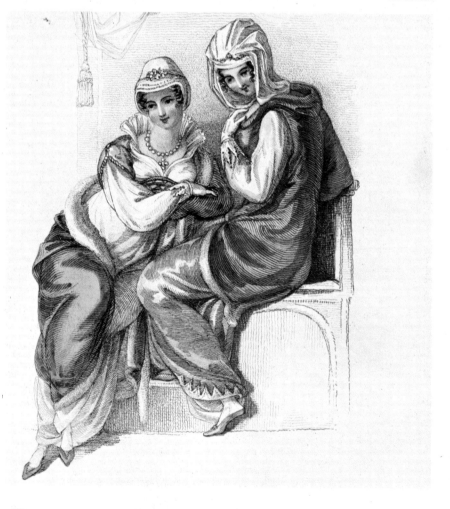

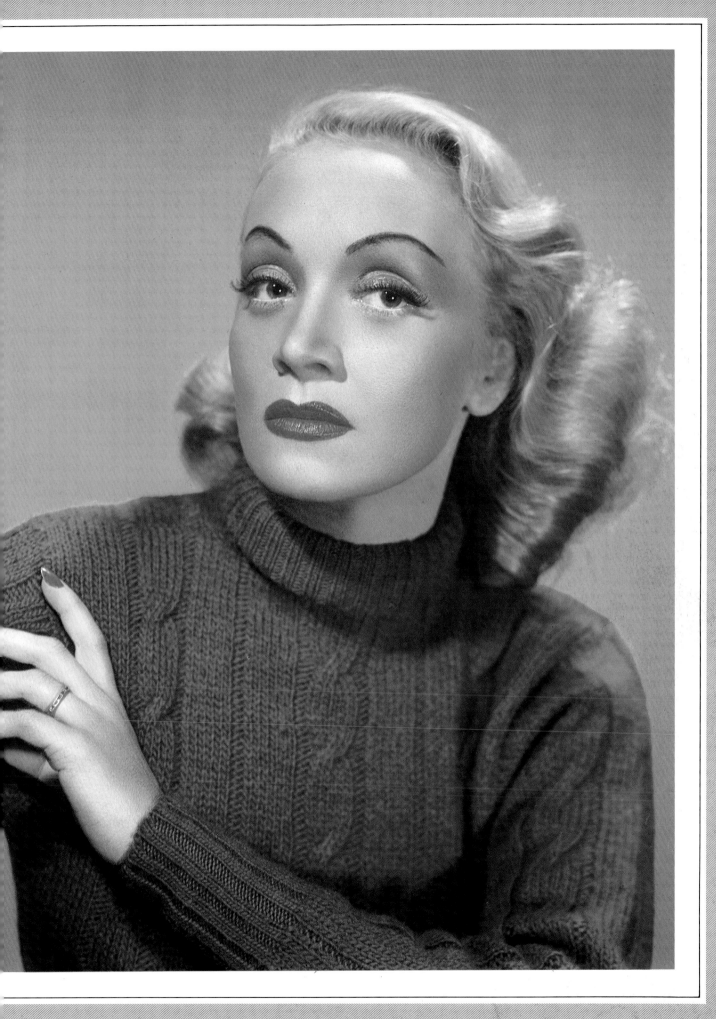

pretty much the same, but its popularity increased in the reign of Charles II, when Nell Gwynn's success with the monarch resulted in well-born ladies copying the exaggerated stage make-up of actresses as part of their daily cosmetic routine. A normal make-up of that period would consist of a face blanched with powder and cheeks dyed with Spanish leather rouge from Seville (a piece of scarlet leather which coloured the skin on application). Blemishes would be covered with pieces of this same leather shaped like stars or crescent moons.

The 18th-century ideal of beauty was a china-doll type of woman with powdered curls and a softly blushing complexion. Very often these fragile little faces hid grotesque realities, as not only had the use of white lead face powder well and truly taken its toll by now, causing headaches, dizziness, constipation and even blindness, but poor diet and insanitary living conditions had also had their effect, and very few fashionable beauties managed to keep their looks much beyond the age of 30. However, none of these appalling symptoms managed to halt the use of white lead as face powder, and the final kiss of death to the fashionable 18th-century complexion was rouge, which included carmine, a rouge blanche made from a white-lead base, vegetable rouge, and a 'serviette rouge', a rag dipped in colouring dye. One strange fashion dictate was the use of mouse skin eyebrows, which were considered the height of elegance. Unfortunately, these did not always stay in place, and it was a familiar sight to see frantic adjustments being made while the owner attempted to remain nonchalant.

There were absolutely no lengths to which an 18th-century woman would not go to attract a husband or lover, and 'beauty' recipes were common, often including such unlikely and unromantic ingredients as frog's

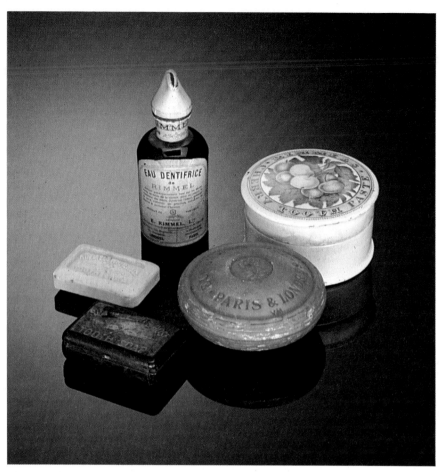

In days of old make-up preparations were crude, home-made and sometimes even lethal. Since the 1930s, when the beauty industry really began to flourish, products have become increasingly sophisticated. Picture courtesy of Rimmel.

blood, leeches and goat's cheese. The next century, however, saw a complete about turn, with the society women of the early 19th century appearing light-boned and pretty. Harmful cosmetic ingredients were replaced by herbs, flowers, vegetable fats and oils. Vegetable rouges were made from red sandalwood, cochineal, brazilwood and saffron mixed with talc. By the mid-19th century, the Victorian ideal of beauty had become an innocent, natural-looking face with a rosebud mouth, dimpled cheeks and small neat features. Rouge and powder were now applied sparingly with a hare's-foot or camel-hair brush, and lip salve was only ever used if lips were chapped.

By the end of the century women had begun to liberate themselves from the demure Victorian look. Rouged cheeks

became more obvious again, and eyes were enhanced with kohl, and lashes thickened with coconut oil and darkened with mascara. The Edwardians preferred a chocolate-box appearance to the previous rather understated prettiness, and once again generous applications of rouge and contrasting chalky white powder became the norm.

Towards the end of the Edwardian era a new breed of women appeared, quite revolutionary by British cosmetic standards. These women, the high-class courtesans, would use make-up in an individual way to suit their own faces, an expertise shared by actresses, whose techniques influenced other ladies of that era. One dancer and actress shaded her features with a mushroom-coloured powder, defining her chin with a light dusting of ter-

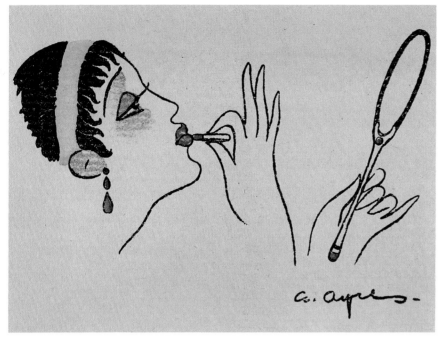

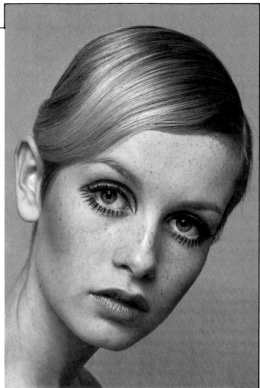

racotta applied with a hare's foot. Her cheeks were tinted with a coral rouge, and the corners of her eyes and nostrils emphasized with dots of red, green or mauve paint.

The outbreak of the First World War saw make-up much more widely used than ever before, as the process of women's emancipation accelerated and the class barriers began to break down. There was no longer any secret about cosmetics, which were even blatantly applied in public. In the 1920s vivid lip colour made its debut, and the two essential tools of any make-up kit were lipstick and eyebrow pencil. Bright colours were used to paint a cupid's-bow shape over the natural form of the mouth, and a thin, arched line was pencilled over eyebrows which had first been extensively plucked. Eyebrow pencils were also used to turn facial moles into beauty spots. Eyelids were coloured for the evening but just glossed with lanolin during the day.

By the 1930s the beauty business had become a thriving industry, make-up had become more refined and colours much more varied. Now magazines gave advice on the use of make-up, and false eyelashes were even used by really daring women. After the Second World War a new image of femininity was created by the world of fashion and beauty, the ideal being one of superficial glamour, with lipsticks and nail varnishes becoming the most popular cosmetics. In the 1950s a cosmetic firm called Gala broke all cosmetic boundaries and introduced a shade of powder and foundation based on yellow and pink colouring ingredients – beige make-up, hitherto undreamed of! This marked the realization that skin tones need not conform to a stereotype, but that each type of complexion could be attractive in its own right. As people could now afford to travel abroad and sunbathe, darker complexions began to be considered attractive, and paler lipsticks were introduced to flatter and complement them. At last attention switched from the lips to the eyes. Exaggerated black lines would be drawn to emphasize the upper lid of the eye and elongate the corners.

The theatrical world continued to influence cosmetic fashion, and English girls, attracted by the Continental type of beauty seen in European films in the early 1960s, would use heavy black eye make-up and pale lipstick to give them

the 'pale and interesting' look seen among French students.

Ever since make-up has grown and flourished to give the refined products and almost endless variety we have at our disposal today. But even so, many of the ingredients used in modern beauty products would be familiar to both ancient Egyptians and to Elizabethans. Talc and rice powder, for instance, still form the basis of face powders, and natural waxes, oils and fats are employed as agents in the manufacture of all-in-one face make-ups. Colouring ingredients are manufactured from basic earth pigments, iron oxides, charcoals and various ochres. But one thing that has changed is that fashion no longer dictates the way a face should look. A myriad of products and techniques are out there to ensure that a woman can bring out the character of her face and make the most of what she has.

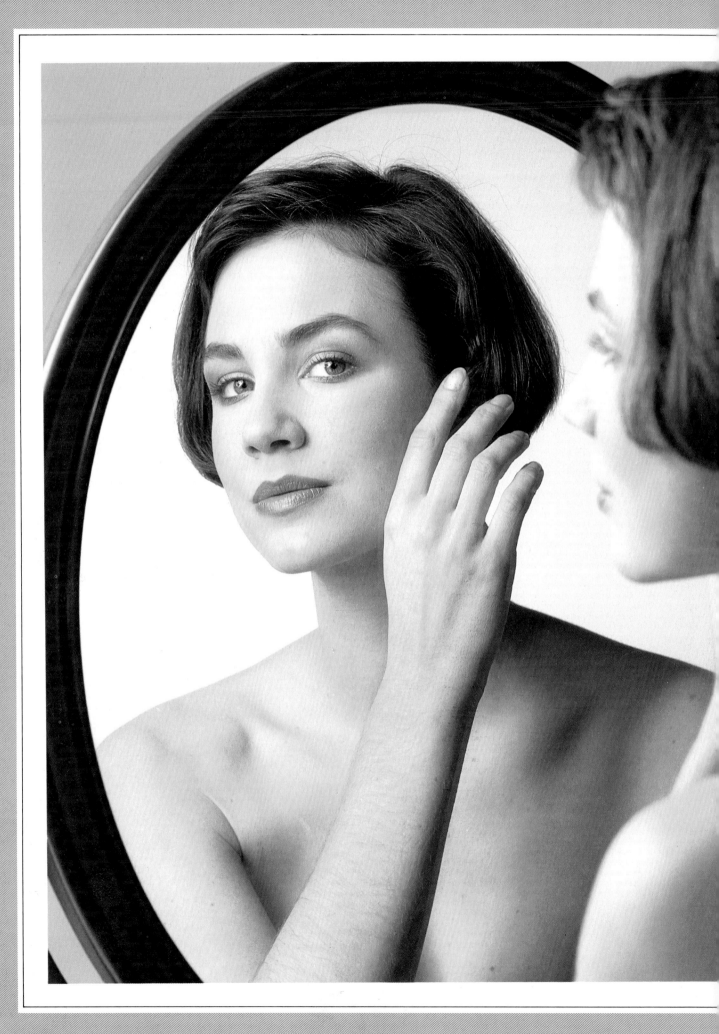

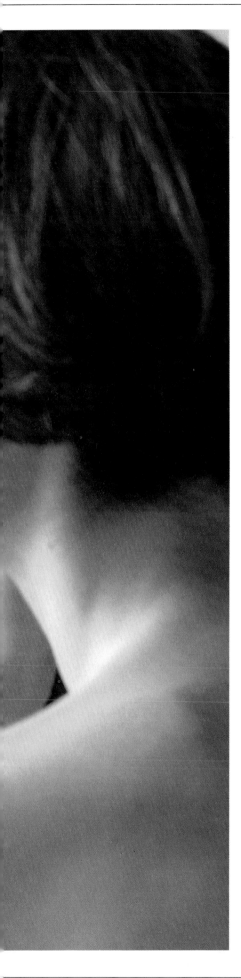

Skin deep

Before we go into greater detail about the application and selection of make-up, it's important to understand more about the 'canvas' on which we are applying it, for no artist can create a successful picture if the work surface is not properly prepared.

Skin is actually a marvellous, almost magical, organ. It's one of the largest of the human body and certainly one of the most efficient. Not only is it the great protector against outside elements, it is also a self-cleaning organ – it clears the waste matter and poisons both from the system and from itself. It even grows, reacts to sensation, and constantly renews itself.

The structure of the skin

The skin is divided into three layers: the epidermis, the corium, or dermis, and the subcutaneous tissue. The outer layer of the skin, the epidermis, is also the thinnest, and although the skin cells can be spotted only through a microscope, they are very active. Twenty to thirty times thicker than the epidermis is the corium, or dermis, which is the true skin, resting on a thick pad of fatty subcutaneous tissue which acts as a kind of shock absorber and insulator for the body. As we have already mentioned, skin acts as a barrier between the organs inside

It is essential to thoroughly know your skin type before you even begin to think about applying make-up. An artist can never apply a palette to the wrong or a dirty canvas! Photography courtesy of Christy Cosmetics.

the body and the world outside, but it does have more specific functions. A healthy skin is soft and elastic, and it protects the body from physical and chemical injury and from bacteria. The sweat glands and blood vessels of the skin's body are like heat regulators, and they keep the body's internal temperature at 98.6 degrees. Blood flows into the vessels to keep the body warm, while the sweat glands act like a cooling system.

The skin is also alert to many sensations and its surface contains a network of nerve endings which enable the body to feel heat, cold, pain and touch. Many people believe that skin is absorbent, but this is not true. Most liquids will not penetrate the skin unless the layers have actually been destroyed in some way, but many gases and volatile substances can easily pass through it.

The epidermis itself, has its own distinct layers. The horny outer layer is made up of several layers of dead, keratinized cells. This layer contains the least amount of water, only 10 to 20 per cent, while the other layers contain 70 per cent. The minute cells of this outer layer are constantly peeled off by things like clothing and bed linen, but the underlying layer is protected by keratin, a very tough and elastic layer of protein. When the water content of the horny outer layer falls below 10 per cent, the skin becomes chapped, and is visibly dry and scaly. Dry skin is not caused by a lack of skin oil, or sebum, but by a lack of moisture. The granular layer of the skin is the strongest in the areas where the lucid layer, a barrier layer

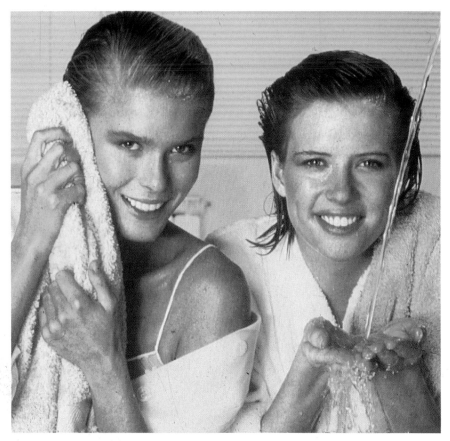

Your beauty régime should be determined by your skin type. Make absolutely certain you know what kind of skin you are buying for, before you start investing in cleansing and moisturizing preparations. Picture courtesy of Vichy.

found on the palms of the hands and soles of the feet, is absent. It protects the body from physical and chemical penetration. The prickle layer is made up of several layers of the epidermal cells that connect four or more keratin or melanin cells. The basal layer of cells lies above the dermis. These cells form keratin and melanin.

Skin types

There are three basic skin types, and knowing which one you have is absolutely crucial, not only for the care of your skin but for your choice of make-up. Many people remain frustrated for years, believing that they are unable to apply make-up properly, when they have just been selecting the wrong product for their skin type. The three basic types are dry, oily and combination. It's fairly easy to

spot your own category, although some people do make the mistake of believing they have dry or oily skin when really it is a combination of both – and this makes a world of difference to any beauty routine. If your skin is oily you will probably be prone to spots, the surface of the skin will appear shiny, and your hair will very likely be oily too. Dry skin appears flaky, while combination skin has an oily centre panel, down the cheeks, chin and forehead, but is dryer elsewhere.

Oily skin

This is often considered a problem, but in fact it is a good skin, easily coaxed to look its best. The pores of an oily skin are constantly active, owing to the hormone balance of the whole body, and it is often the case that people with an abundance of energy have oily skin, the hormones being actively related to general physique. Oily

skin is more common amongst young people, because it is during this development period that sebaceous secretion tends to be over-productive, causing dilated pores and a shiny appearance.

Provided it is allowed to flow freely and not accumulate, oil is actually an asset to the skin, as it protects it and preserves it against ageing. But if the oil accumulates and then congeals, it forms a blockage over the opening of the pores, causing loaded pores and blackheads. Despite this, the skin still tries to excrete waste matter and oil, and nature reacts by causing the pores to dilate. This leads to enlarged, open pores. The stale excretion can also become an irritant which then becomes infected, hence spots and pimples. The very worst thing you can ever do to a spot is squeeze it, indeed, a good general rule for skin care is to touch your face as little as possible, if ever. Oily skin appears to be thicker than dry skin, but it does bruise easily, and each time you press too hard trying to remove a blackhead a mark will remain. There are fatty beads underneath the spots which are housed in capsules under the bottom layer of the skin. When you squeeze a spot you crush these beads and release oil in the tissues that the sebaceous glands cannot cope with. This all gets stale and stuck in the pores, and even more blemishes will occur, so remember, *leave those spots alone.* The best way to deal with a blemished skin is from within, so watch your diet, as greasy foods will take their toll.

Travelling, tension and fatigue are all enemies of skin which is prone to blemishes. Wash the skin frequently with soap and water. This dries the skin and causes mild peeling, which in turn helps to eliminate plug formation. Remove excess oil with an astringent. As a preventive measure it is a good idea to exfoliate regularly. Exfoliation is the removal of the dead skin flakes that form every day on the surface of the skin, and it allows a better-looking skin to show. However, never go overboard with excessive use and, if you notice any redness or irritation, then stop. Oil-free make-up should be applied to oily skin, but be careful here, because oil-free does not necessarily mean the same thing as water-based, which is a combination of water plus oil. A gel or a powder blusher are good choices for oily skin, but if your skin is oily and your powder blusher blotches, this is a sure sign that you have selected the wrong foundation, as it will not sit properly on the wrong base.

Acne is a severe form of blemished skin which needs careful handling. It is quite common and not a serious disease, but it is disfiguring and can lead to serious scarring. It usually occurs at puberty, when the activity of endocrine glands increases. These glands secrete hormones that affect various parts of the body including the sebaceous glands of the skin. During adolescence the sebaceous glands enlarge and become active, and this enlargement and the excess of oily material that the glands produce are the essential features of acne. While most of the oil produced by the glands reaches the surface, some may be pushed back in the ducts of the large oil glands, producing blackheads and white-heads which may eventually break through the walls of the ducts to become the pimples and boil-like lesions.

As many as 80 per cent of all teenagers have some degree of acne, and it can linger into the 20s. Even some 30-year-olds who have previously never had a spot in their lives can suddenly fall foul of it. Acne is not caused by dirt, but washing your face with soap and hot water three or four times a day helps to control the oiliness. Supervision by a doctor will help ensure minimal skin involvement and scarring, and some doctors advise using soap that contains an antiseptic to decrease bacteria on the skin's surface. Avoid inflaming your skin through exposing it to excessive humidity, greasy cosmetics, some varieties of the contraceptive pill or too much stress. And once again – *don't touch.*

Oily skin is the bane of many a young person's life and it is a sad fact of life that this skin type is more prone to spots. The situation can be eased though, with a good, healthy diet. Picture (*right*) courtesy of Almay and (*below*) Schwarzkopf.

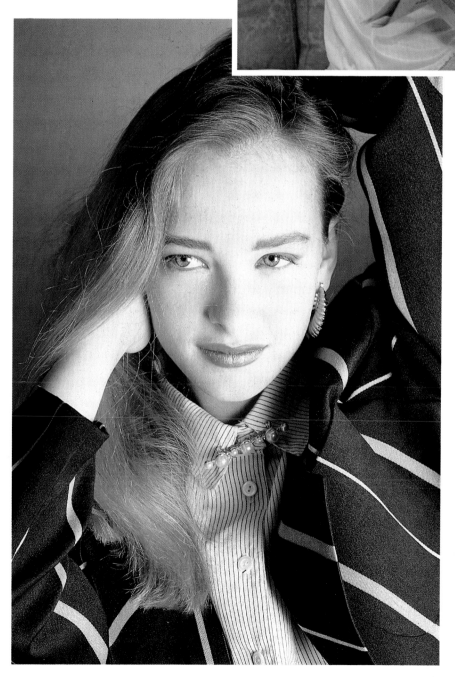

Dry skin

Dryness of the skin is primarily due to loss of water from the skin's horny outer layer and insufficient movement of moisture upward from lower tissue layers. Dry skin has no visible pores, is often traced with superficial wrinkles, and is inclined to age prematurely. A good graphic description of dry skin is one which feels a size or two too small for your face. The aim is to coax it into behaving normally and to re-establish a fresh, healthy bloom. Regular cleansing is as important with this skin type as with any other, but you may prefer using a cleansing cream to soap and water, as water used too hot and too often will have a drying effect. It is important to moisturize dry skin regularly, but do be careful when selecting your product. Remember that no matter how many magical ingredients a moisturizer may contain, nothing can actually penetrate through to your skin beyond the horny outer layer. Your skin cannot be fed from the outside, only from within.

Excessive dryness is one of the changes in skin, along with wrinkling and the brown spots of hyper-pigmentation that we associate with ageing. These changes are directly or indirectly due to the ultraviolet rays of sunlight. They begin early on in life, and can be exaggerated if a particularly fair-skinned person has to live in a sunny climate. Avoiding the sunshine and using protective barrier creams from childhood are the only ways of slowing down these changes, for they cannot be reversed. Exotic rejuvenating creams can only offer temporary relief from excessive dryness by softening and smoothing fine lines and rough skin. When a face ages its contours change, the natural lines on the face and neck deepen and become more obvious, the skin becomes slack and sags into pouches, and the colour changes. In a fine-textured, older skin, the slower rate of sebaceous secretion is thought to play a major role in the ageing process. The oily liquid produced by the sebaceous glands contains fatty acids, lipids and cellular matter which help protect the skin from bacteria and external drying elements. Although there is no reversing this process, it has been observed that women who have always followed a good skin-care routine do retain a more

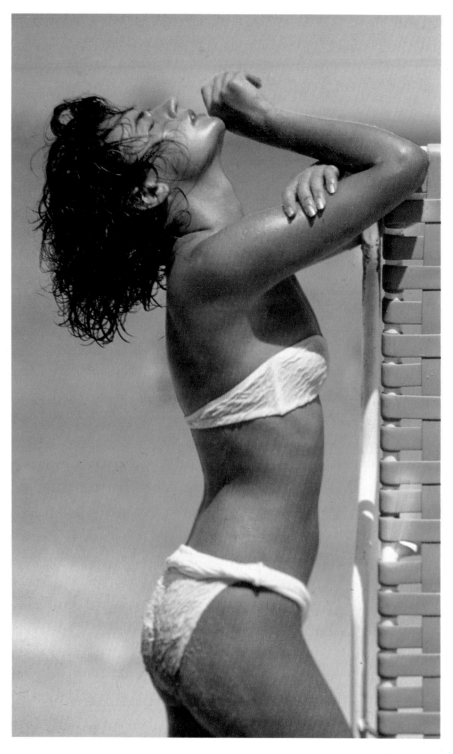

Excessive dryness in the skin is associated with ageing and it is true that too much sunshine can have an adverse effect on the skin, often causing it to wrinkle before its time. Enjoy being out in the sunshine but always wear a protective cream as this picture (above) from the Boots System I Range shows. *Right:* Learn how to treat your skin kindly and adapt to it as it ages and you will most certainly mature gracefully. Picture courtesy of Schwarzkopf.

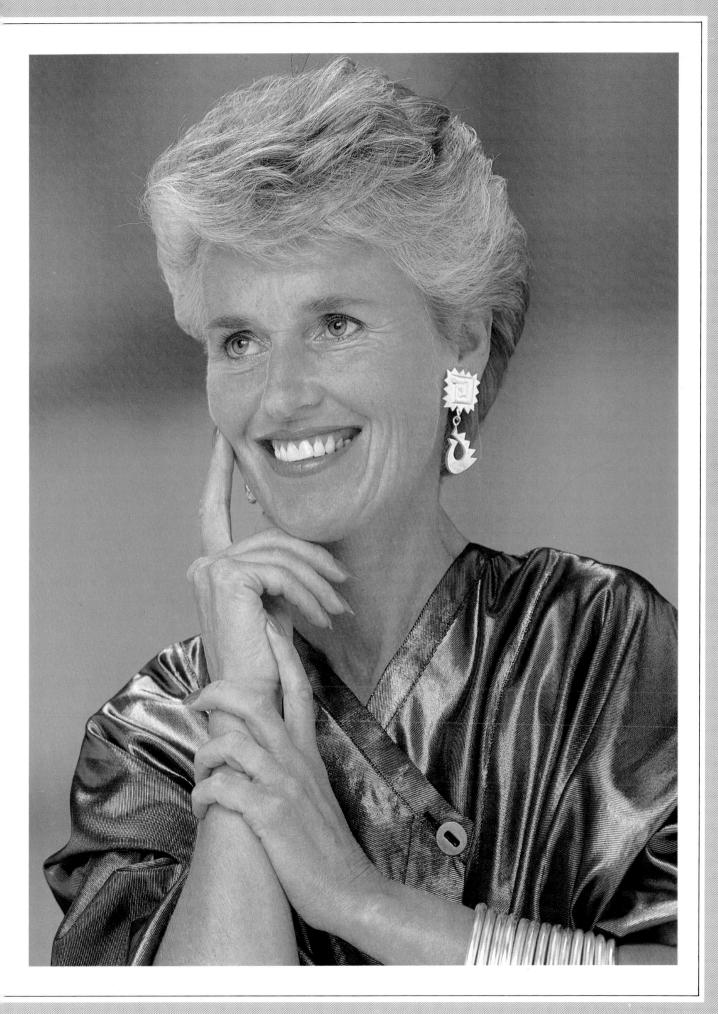

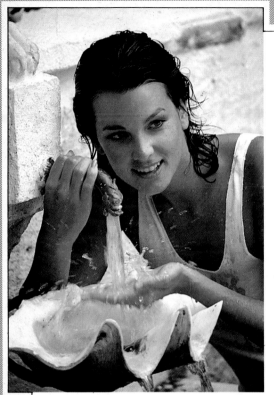

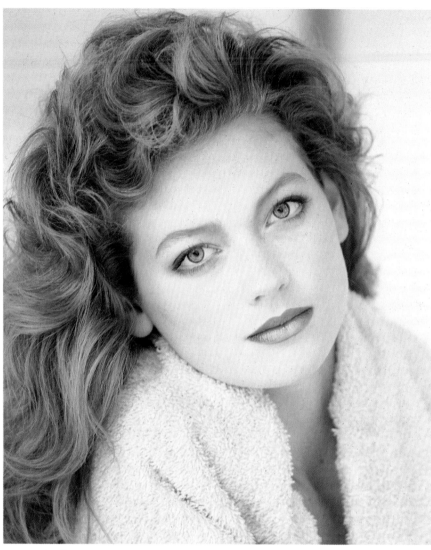

To refresh your face, you may like to splash it with ice cold water in the morning, as illustrated by Mary Quant Cosmetics above. *Right:* Creamier cleansing and moisturizing products may be necessary for drier skin to achieve a fresh-faced glow. Picture courtesy of Almay.

youthful appearance, probably because they have been stimulating the sebaceous secretion level. So once again, a good skin-care routine, no matter how simple, is all-important from an early age.

Bags and dark circles under the eyes are other signs of ageing, as some underlying eye tissues and muscles are lost as a person grows older, and the lower lids tend to fall in folds. Underlying fat pushes through weakened muscles, causing the baggy tissue to balloon out. Dark circles occur when the blood that passes through the large veins to the surface of the eyelid actually shows through the skin, producing a bluish-black tint. This can happen at various times in life, but the discoloration becomes more obvious and permanent as a person gets older.

Combination skin

Proper care of combination skin requires flexible use of facial cosmetics. Washing with a moderately drying soap two or three times a day and the use of a non-greasy cleanser will decrease oiliness in the centre areas of the face. Excessive dryness on the sides of cheeks, temples and eyelids may be relieved by lubricating cream, used sparingly, morning and evening. If excessive oiliness persists, an astringent solvent may be used two or three times daily on forehead, nose and chin. No single cosmetic will care for all skin areas of people with combination skin, so remain open-minded about what you use and how you use it. It may be necessary to use two different types of foundation, one for the dry and one for the oily areas of the face.

Normal skin

So far we have only discussed the problem, but there is such a thing as the ideal skin, and women who have it never complain about it! Beautiful skin has no blemishes, roughness or peeling. It has a coloration that appears uniform. The upper layers of an unclogged skin will have a translucence which reflects the light. But this skin type needs as much loving care and attention as any other if it is to maintain its good looks.

Selecting the product

Selecting the right product for any skin type is half the battle. Choose your products slowly and wisely. When you go into a store to buy any cosmetics, take a good long look around. Before you buy anything you should have the product explained and, if possible, demonstrated to you, so look for a consultant who is busy servicing customers and whose counter isn't cluttered. A busy consultant is one who obviously takes the time to explain the products, and an uncluttered counter will give her the work space she needs. The most expensive brands aren't necessarily the best, but the chances are that more research has gone into them and that they will contain more lasting qualities.

Cosmetic counters laden with creams, lotions and potions which claim to delay the ageing process often resemble chemistry laboratories, and the mind can boggle. The most common of these products are likely to be soluble collagen, hormone creams and tissue extracts. Soluble collagen products are said to increase the skin's capacity to retain fluid, improve its elasticity and therefore provide a more youthful appearance. Hormone creams satisfy the need for oestrogen on the skin of women of post-menopausal age where the natural oestrogen level has decreased, and are also claimed to have the effect of improving the skin's softness, smoothness and elasticity. Tissue extracts are somewhat controversial skin-care preparations as they are obtained from the epidermis, ovaries and placenta of young animals (sheep in particular) which are rich in nutrients and vitamins. They are said to nourish and hydrate ageing skin tissue by increasing capillary circulation and stimulating the metabolism of the skin.

The method of treatment may be a 10-day plan, with the serum extracts individually presented in ampoule form, or they may be a range of products for all aspects of a skin-care routine. The most usual is a treatment to be applied at home over a period of about 10 days to three weeks, with some rest periods included in between.

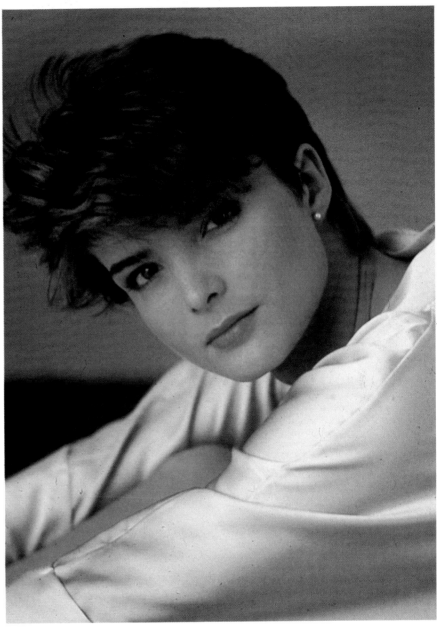

The more time and effort you apply to getting your skin as flawless as possible, the easier it will be to put on your make-up and the more attractive the end result will be. Picture courtesy of Dior.

I have to remain sceptical about the claims and effects of any of these products, since I firmly believe that nothing can penetrate and nourish that dead top layer of skin. But having said that, I must confess that my mother is a great fan of exotic moisturizing and nourishing preparations and, although she is over 60, her skin looks at least 15 years younger, with a light, youthful glow. Her beauty ideals have rubbed off on me and, since the age of 11, I have taken care of my skin, finding simple beauty routines to suit my changing, maturing skin type, and I too have been told my skin looks young for its age. But I remain unconvinced as to whether this success is due to the actual products we have used (and there have been so many of them between us that it would be impossible to pinpoint any in particular) or the fact that we simply look after our skin at all times, detect any faults at an early stage, and really believe in ourselves and the way we look.

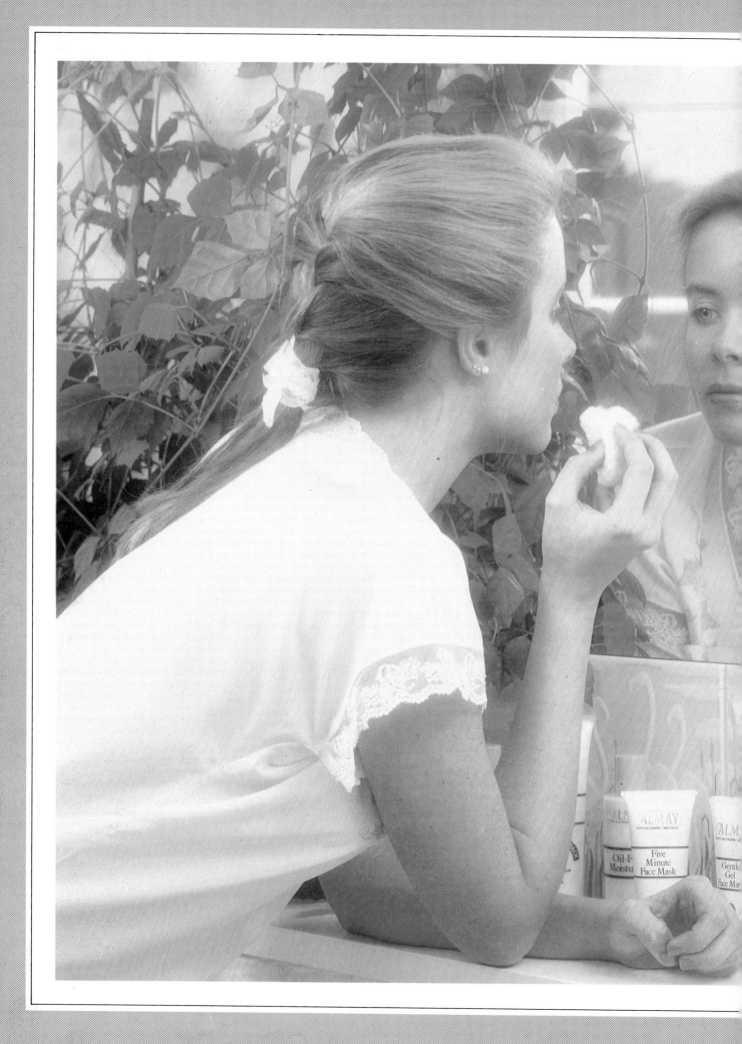

Clean supreme

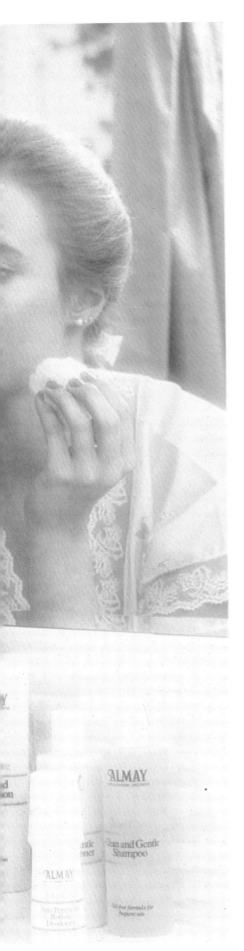

There are thousands of skin-care cosmetics on the market and it's easy to fall foul of good marketing jargon, pretty packaging and magical ingredients which, once home, don't do the trick. This can be an expensive and time-wasting hobby, so if you really are in doubt about your skin type or think you have a problem you're not sure how to solve, then seek out a skin-care specialist or a dermatologist for expert advice. When selecting your cleansing preparations ask yourself these questions. Will it remove all my make-up thoroughly? Is it really suitable for my skin type? Does it have the correct texture for easy application? Does it feel pleasant on my skin? Can I afford it?

The following is a brief analysis of some of the cleansing products available, as knowing how they vary, will help you to do the battle of the beauty counter.

Cleansing products

Cleansing milks are emulsions which are made of different forms of water and oil. Cleansing milk is essentially a diluted cleansing cream, which may have an appearance of actual milk or be jelly-like in consistency. In either case the product will appear to be light and grease-free. The more liquid

The vast array of cleansing preparations on the market can be bewildering. You should match the product to your own skin type and then make sure when cleansing that every last trace of dirt and grime are removed. Picture courtesy of Almay.

and thin in consistency a product is, the higher is the chance that it contains more water than oil, less effective for removing heavy or oily based make-up. The detergent element in many cleansing milks, though making them effective in removing surface bacteria and oily blockages from the skin on a young, make-up free face, can be drying on mature or sensitive skins, which need cleansing milks with a higher oil content. You'll know whether or not a cleansing milk has a high fluid content by the way it feels on your skin. It will feel cool and pleasant to use and will leave the skin free from oil after removal.

The middle range of cleansing milks, sometimes sold as emulsions, have many uses and suit many skin types. They have a high proportion of oil to water, have less or no detergent and are quickly and effectively capable of removing all traces of make-up. Products for dry and sensitive skins are available within this group of cleansing milks, and these can be recognized by their jelly-like consistency and the glossy appearance they assume on application to the skin. The skin will take on a slight sheen after the removal of this type of product.

Heavy cleansing milks have a high oil-to-water proportion, feel more oily on the skin and take on a very definite sheen when applied to the skin. They do not drag the skin and can act as a lubricant when the surface is dry. But they will leave an oily film after removal, which makes it necessary to thoroughly tone all the facial skin afterwards.

Cleansing creams are the most efficient cleansers, and particularly suit dry, stretched, dehydrated or maturing skin types. They dissolve make-up rapidly so that the skin does not have to be over-manipulated, which could cause over-stimulation of the surface capillaries.

Liquifying cleansing creams are really designed for the fast removal of particularly heavy make-up, the sort worn for television or the stage. They are the only creams that are not based on a water-in-oil formulation, being made up of oily materials only. This makes them suitable for dry, loose skins, which may benefit from the feeling of lubrication left after cleansing.

Soapless cleansers and *complexion soaps* are a form of soap which do not leave the skin feeling taut, as normal soap sometimes does. For oily or blemished skins that are also sensitive, these cleansers are kinder in action, and can be used frequently without irritation resulting. Soapless cleansers come in liquid, semi-liquid, tube or soap-bar form, and they are designed to deep-cleanse an already clean skin rather than remove make-up.

Cleansing lotions have a degreasing effect on sebaceous material present on the skin's surface, and so are useful in the case of oily or blocked skins. They will leave skin with a stripped feeling after use, but rather than relying on them as total cleansers it is best to use them as fresheners on the skin once make-up has been thoroughly removed or as a pick-me-up on make-up free skin during the day.

Pore or cleansing grains, very popular these days, are actually detergent chips, which are made into a gritty paste in the palm of the hand with a few drops of water, and used like an abrasive rub to free oily blockage. The paste is worked into the skin, kept moist and rinsed off after a few

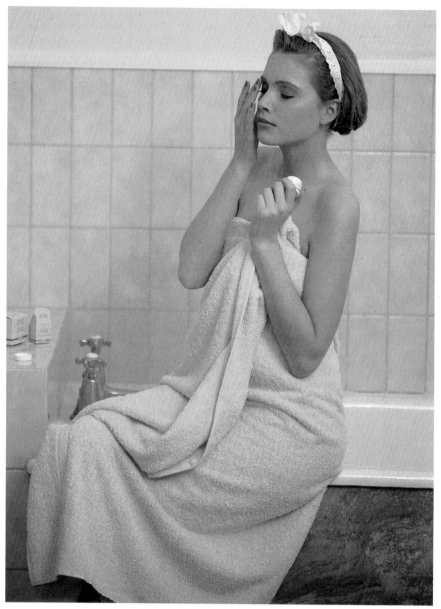

Cleansing creams are particularly efficient as they dissolve dirt rapidly. There are many different types of cleansing creams though so read about the product in detail or, better still, consult the manufacturer for advice. Picture courtesy of Almay.

minutes. Used carefully, these can be helpful in the prevention of blocked pores, but you should seek advice as to their use, as it may be necessary to apply them daily, weekly or monthly depending on the degree of oiliness.

Cleansing routines

For a long time the cleanse, tone and moisturize routine theory was plugged so hard that it was considered essential. But you will see from the above list of cleansers

that any beauty régime depends on the skin type and major cleanser used. Ask any make-up free women whether she is wearing cosmetics and she will say no, without thinking of her moisturizer. This is, of course, a cosmetic also, but its use has become so automatic that people don't regard it as such any more.

It may not be necessary to tone your skin at all, and certainly it is not always necessary to moisturize it. Sometimes a very fine spray of water is all that's needed to replace moisture lost from the

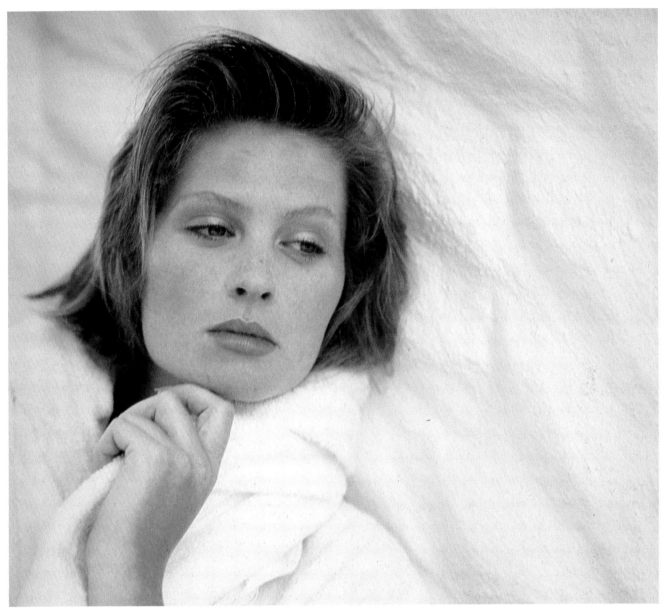

Arguments for various beauty routines are strong, but do remember that products are designed to work together so it is often wise to stick to just one brand. Picture courtesy of the No 7 Special Collection.

skin during the day and, if the skin is particularly oily, the last thing it wants is a heavy, greasy cream which has to be worked in, stimulating those already busy sebaceous glands. Some cosmetic manufacturers now list exfoliation (the removal of the dead flakes that form every day on the skin's surface) as a top beauty priority. It is arguable whether exfoliation is not just another name for the cleanse, tone and moisturize routine, and that perhaps the right cleansing agents, used on a daily basis, would have the same effect, but it does help the skin take on

that lovely, translucent, eventoned look we all struggle to achieve. It is also a relatively quick, easy and enjoyable way of treating ourselves on a regular basis.

Basically, the kind of products you opt for are very much a matter of personal taste, but remember that ranges are designed to be complementary to one another, so research your manufacturer carefully and then stick to one range of products. Expert advice is important with product selection: you might, for instance, have oily or greasy skin and like to feel it

stripped clean and free from oil, but in doing so you could be stimulating the sebaceous glands further. So look for a consultant and examine her own appearance. If she seems sloppy or badly made up, take this as a reflection on her attitude to work. She's hardly likely to want to spend the time analyzing your skin type and problems if she can't be bothered to spend time on herself. And don't allow yourself to get trapped by a hard-sell technique. A good consultant should at least appear to be more concerned about you than her commission.

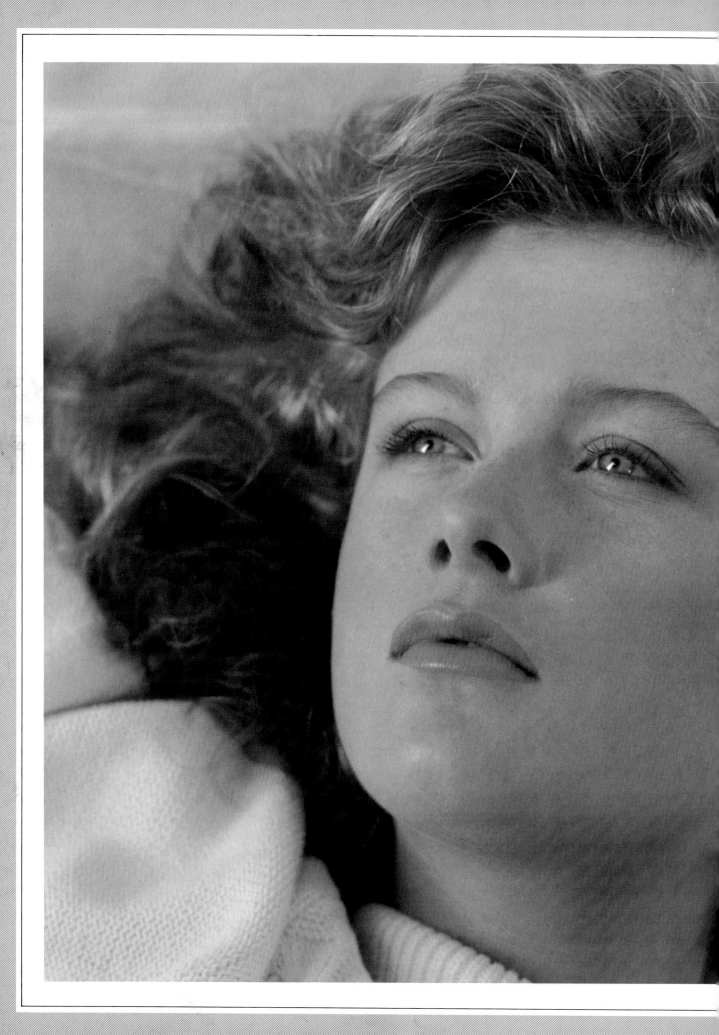

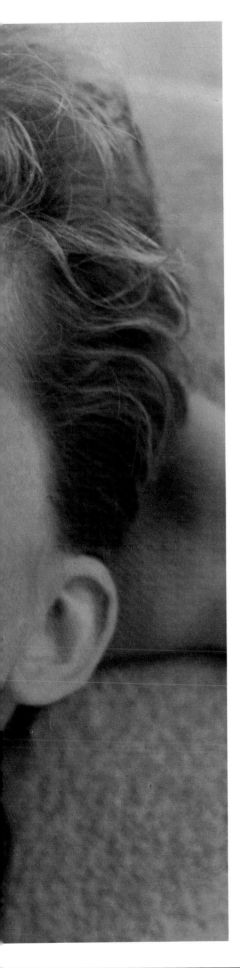

A tidy face is a happy face

Eyebrows

Having established your skin type and made sure your face is as glowing and blemish-free as it can be, you may think you are all ready to start with the make-up palette. Think again. Take another long, hard look at that naked face in the mirror. Are there any unsightly, unwanted hairs that could be banished but that you've chosen to ignore before? Are your eyebrows too thin or too bushy, too straggly or just plain out of shape? Your eyebrows frame the face and help give it character and balance, so if they've always been a problem to you before, take a proper, analytical look at them. If you are taking the trouble to read this book you must truly want to look your best, so why not give a little extra attention to your eyebrows? They can completely ruin the most perfectly made-up face if they are untidy or are simply uneven!

Nothing looks worse than eyebrows which have been severely plucked or totally obliterated. Eyebrows are at their best fairly thick and well trimmed, but not so 'natural' that they either meet in the middle or leave no space on which to apply eye make-up. For most of us a little bit of trimming is necessary.

Eyebrows should be neat and tidy with enough space for a little creative make-up. When you first start, pluck them with caution, if you are too ruthless they'll just pale into insignificance! Picture courtesy of Almay.

Eyebrow shaping

A good way of seeing whether your brows are in good shape is to place a slim pencil in a straight line at the side of your nose. The eyebrow should start at this point and not before it. Any hairs on the other side of the pencil, near the bridge of the nose, need to go. Now measure a 45-degree angle from the outside corner of the eye. This is where the eyebrow should end and, once again, any straggly hairs on the other side of the pencil need to be eliminated. Hold the pencil parallel to the nose along the outside edge of your iris. Ideally, this is where the arch of the eyebrow should be, although I do feel that if nature has endowed you with a well-shaped brow anyway and you are satisfied with the space on which you have to put your make-up you shouldn't be too ruthless with the tweezers.

Eyebrow plucking

If you've never plucked your brows before, then it might be a good idea to have them done professionally for the first few times, as some people do find the process painful. But I believe, in general, that it is far better to 'pluck up' courage and be in control of your own destiny than to let a beautician take out brows that you won't know are missing until it's too late. On your first attempt, pluck only a few at a time and take a fresh look every day to see how they are progressing and whether the shape is right.

Once they are the shape you want they obviously need keeping in trim on a regular basis. Some people pluck their brows only once a week, but I feel that no harm can be done by at least checking them for any noticeable regrowth every morning in the mirror before you think about applying your make-up.

Before you start to pluck your brows make sure you have the best possible light, either natural daylight or illuminated magnification. In addition to your mirror and tweezers you'll need some gentle antiseptic solution – which will have a cooling effect as well as guarding against any risk of infection – and some cotton wool. Start between the brows first, removing any stray hairs from the inner corners. Now support and stretch the skin with one hand while you start to work under the brow with the other. Pluck only in the direction in which the hair grows, and use the antiseptic solution as often as you need to. This will help cool and soothe the skin, which is bound to be irritated and to react to such a disturbance.

Now look above the brow towards the temple in case there are any stray hairs there. Have a rest and take a look at one brow before you move on to the other to make sure it's the shape you want it to be. Remember to work slowly and steadily. You want to avoid ending up with eyebrows which are too highly arched, look too furrowed or are too thin. It's only too easy to pluck them out, but if the end result is disastrous you'll have to wait for them to grow back again, which is an untidy and tedious business. If your brows are really bushy and you've never showed them a pair of tweezers before, just pluck a few hairs at a time over a period of two or three weeks. That way you'll get used to the feel of plucking your eyebrows and become accustomed to your new trimmed look.

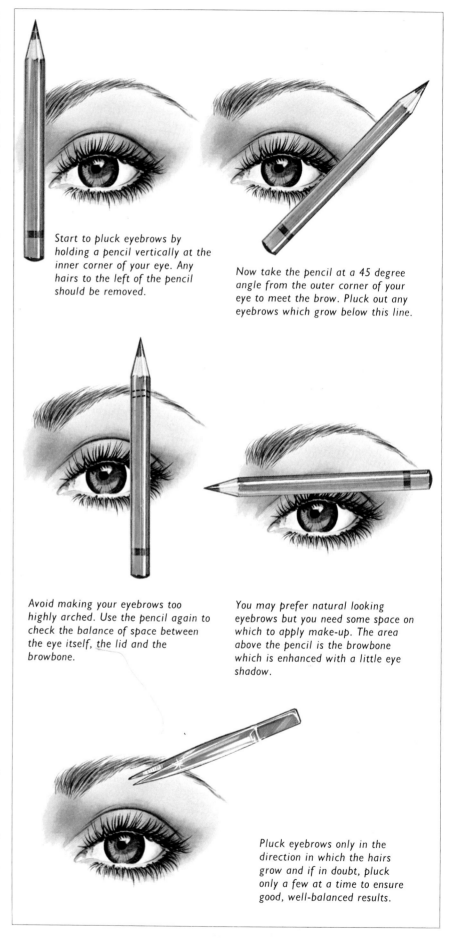

Start to pluck eyebrows by holding a pencil vertically at the inner corner of your eye. Any hairs to the left of the pencil should be removed.

Now take the pencil at a 45 degree angle from the outer corner of your eye to meet the brow. Pluck out any eyebrows which grow below this line.

Avoid making your eyebrows too highly arched. Use the pencil again to check the balance of space between the eye itself, the lid and the browbone.

You may prefer natural looking eyebrows but you need some space on which to apply make-up. The area above the pencil is the browbone which is enhanced with a little eye shadow.

Pluck eyebrows only in the direction in which the hairs grow and if in doubt, pluck only a few at a time to ensure good, well-balanced results.

Eyebrow and eyelash tinting

Eyebrow and eyelash tinting is another way of enhancing what nature has already provided you with and of giving your 'total look' something of a head start. I particularly like to have my eyelashes tinted in the summer so that if I feel like having a day without make-up my eyes don't look too insignificant. Kits can be bought which enable you to tint your eyelashes at home, but I would always advise you to let a professional take over here. It's a messy and frustrating business to do at home and anything to do with the eyes and chemicals should best be left to those who know their business, just in case there is some kind of reaction.

Eyelash tinting is probably more popular than eyebrow tinting. Well-shaped eyebrows usually look best left in their own natural colour, but eyelashes are usually much lighter than the brows and often need a little help. This can, of course, be left to mascara, which is quite adequate, but tinting can help emphasize the lashes by intensifying their colour. You can usually choose between black, blue, grey and brown, but be sure to strike a nice, complementary balance between the lashes and the rest of your colouring. Blue, I think, looks a little too false, and grey often too pale, but you don't want your lashes coloured so strongly that they appear harsh. A word of warning before you start. Although modern tints are mainly of vegetable origin, they rely on a peroxide solution to activate them, so if your eyes are likely to be irritated by this, if you have sensitive eyes or are prone to conjunctivitis, then eyelash tinting is not for you.

Superfluous hair

The lip and chin are other areas of the face which are best freed of superfluous hair before make-up is applied. Some of us are so fair that

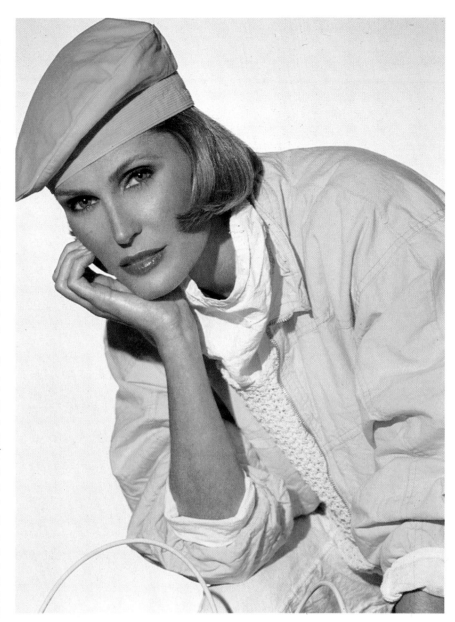

A healthy, well-balanced look like this one may appear completely natural, but it has been given a little help along the way. Get your face in good order and your make-up will glide on all the more easily. Photograph courtesy of Clinique.

the fine hairs in these places hardly show at all and we can go through life ignoring them, but for those of us with darker colouring they are really best waxed away. This is another salon treatment, but a necessary one – I cannot repeat often enough how important it is to have a clean canvas on which to work before you even think of applying make-up. Once you've got your skin and face in perfect shape it will take very little effort to keep them looking good and, like your make-up, will really work wonders to help boost your self-confidence.

Waxing, of course, is only a temporary solution to superfluous hair growth, but it does produce good and instant results which last for between three and six weeks, depending on how quickly it takes your new hairs to grow. If you have particularly fine hairs which regrow quickly or stubborn, strong hairs with a coarse texture, you are probably better off opting for a more permanent form of hair removal like electrolysis, but your beautician is the best person to consult about this.

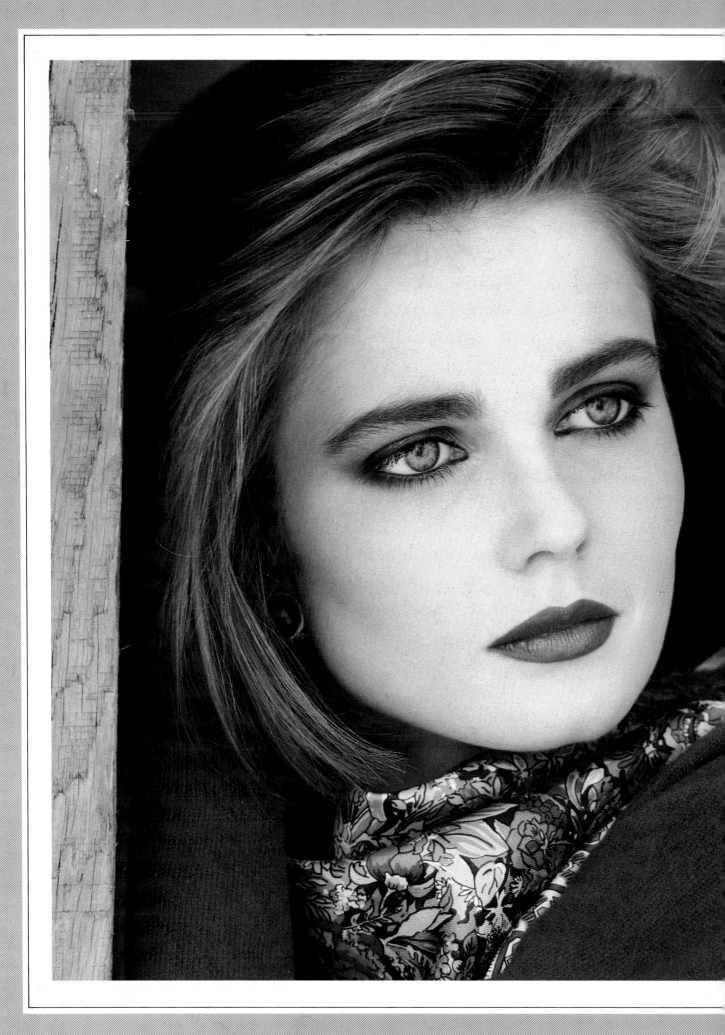

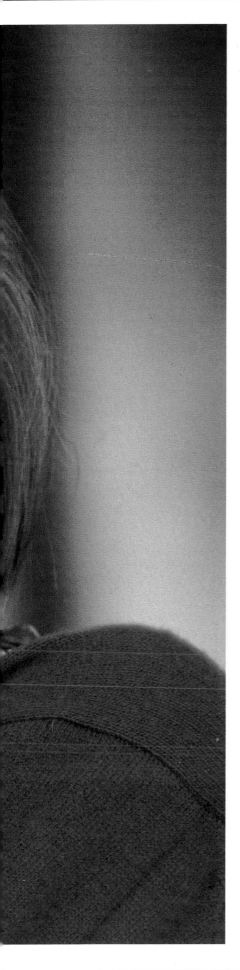

Countdown to make-up

Seeing what is available

The time during which you are busy perfecting your skin-care routine is a good one to start exploring make-up possibilities. Look around at the various brands in magazines and department stores. Compare prices, colour ranges, packaging and presentation, overall quality and consultants. Think long and hard about what you want out of your make-up and how you want to look – or rather, how you see yourself. Your make-up should be a projection of your personality, and a way of communicating, even to total strangers, what kind of a person you are. Remember that you've got to be able to apply your make-up with ease in order to carry it off confidently, so avoid cosmetics which are presented in a way which might prove awkward for you to handle.

Once you have achieved the look which you feel is right for you, you should be able to put on your face in 20 minutes and you don't want to be fiddling around with fancy packaging when you should be on the way to work. Think about the kind of clothes you wear, their colours and style. If you wear lots of creams and russets, for example, you'll want

In the same way that your wardrobe is divided into seasons and different colours, so too should your make-up. Colours are designed to complement one another – and you. Max Factor created this russet and cream look.

to stick to make-up in the more earthy colours rather than bright blues and greens. Look at your own colouring. Does your hair tend to go blonder and your skin darker in summer? If so, you'll probably need two make-up 'wardrobes'.

Take a look at the service that each manufacturer is offering you. Look for a brand which doesn't discontinue its lines quickly. There's nothing more infuriating than finding something which suits you so perfectly it becomes vital to you, only to discover that when it needs renewing it isn't being stocked anymore. Although it can be a good idea to experiment with make-up, I am also a firm believer in sticking with a product if it is absolutely right for you. Finally, think about your budget. There is nothing wrong with the less expensive brands, and they are particularly useful when it comes to eye make-up. You don't need to have more than two or three colours in your eye shadow collection to start with, but when you do want to experiment the cheaper brands enable you to do so without straining your bank balance. When it comes to selecting foundation and blusher, though, opt for the brands which offer a consultancy service. I see so many people wandering around with orange faces or make-up so thick it is almost theatrical and I know it's because they've just picked a product off the counter or asked for one they've seen advertised without checking to see whether it's right for them. Manufacturers like Elizabeth Arden, Dior, Lancôme, Charles of the Ritz, Revlon, Almay and Estée Lauder all offer consultancy services. Clinique go two steps further, with their own computer which taps out your skin type and once you are registered as a Clinique customer, your card is kept on file. This records all your skin details so that if the consultant does change, her successor will already know exactly what your needs are.

A point must be made here about cleanliness when it comes to buying make-up. You shouldn't be expected to test from a lipstick which has probably been used by many people before you. Lipstick should be applied to a cotton bud and then given to you to try. Cotton wool should also be used at the sales counter when customers are experimenting with blushers and powders.

Storage space

Think about where you are going to keep your make-up. I don't beleve that it should be necessary to touch up make-up during the day. One good application should be enough to see you through till early evening (though people with deep-set eyes can 'lose' their eyeshadow, and may need to renew it), and continuously piling on more only makes it look obtrusive. For that reason I don't think anyone needs to keep several complete sets of make-up, one at home, one in the handbag or one at work is not necessary.

Lipstick and powder are all that you'll find in my handbag, even if I am going out straight from work. I will make allowances, however, for the keen disco dancers or night clubbers amongst you. Nightbirds probably do feel they will need a little more definition of colour around the eyes, so I will forgive them using a little eyeshadow and extra mascara!

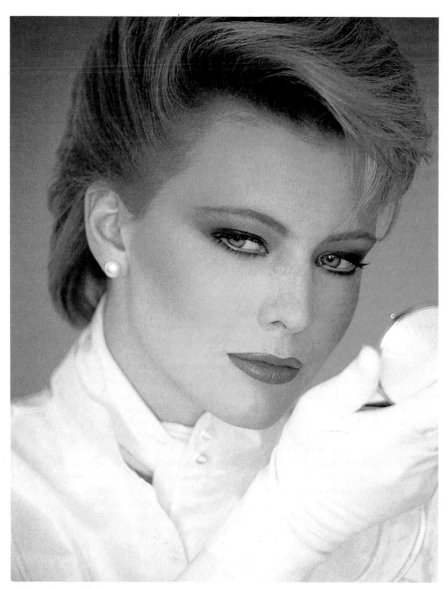

To achieve a make-up with as flawless a finish as this one from Mary Quant, you must look for the best colours and cosmetics to suit you and your lifestyle and then think about a convenient place to store them.

If you have the space then a small drawer in which to keep your make-up is ideal, as this will ensure that it remains clean, dry and dust free. Separate the cosmetics so that eye shadows, lipsticks, foundations, etc, are all in their own places. This way you'll be able to go directly to them. Try and keep your make-up near or at the place where you'll actually be putting it on. This should, wherever possible, be near a window which provides good, natural sunlight in the morning. If you have to resort to artificial lighting try and go out at some time during the day, even if you have to wait until lunchtime, so that you can get a good look at yourself in daylight. Artificial light tends to make your face look paler than it actually is, so your face may need correcting. Also, keep in or near your drawer make-up aids like cotton wool, cotton buds, tissues, a good mirror and tweezers – to keep those eyebrows in check.

Make-up toolkit

Now that you have decided where you are going to store your make-up kit you may think you are all set to go, but there is another essential – tools. Half the secret of a beautifully made-up face is in its skilful application, and the right brushes will not only help your cosmetics to stay on and last longer, but will also feel good to use. They are the best possible way of ensuring a slow and gradual build-up of make-up because they help you to regulate the amount of cosmetics you use.

Long-handled, natural bristle brushes are really the best. Long handles make application easier, and bristle is better than nylon, as the strands of nylon brushes have a tendency to fall out. It is infuriating to have to spend five minutes plucking single strands from your lip brush out of your newly made-up lips! Take care of your tools as well. Good brushes are not cheap, so you want them to last, which they will do provided you handle them properly. For a start, don't let the make-up clog the brushes too much before washing them. The best thing really is to wash them every night. Dangle them gently in a bowl of tepid, soapy water, rinse them thoroughly in lukewarm water and then carefully smooth them back into shape. They are best left to dry naturally, overnight if possible, with the bristles pointing upwards. All this seems a bit long-winded when you haven't even started any making-up yet, but it is important to do your homework first.

Basic make-up kit
The following is a checklist of what a basic make-up kit needs so make sure you have it all.

Foundation. You might need two here, especially if you have a combination skin (see p. 24) or if

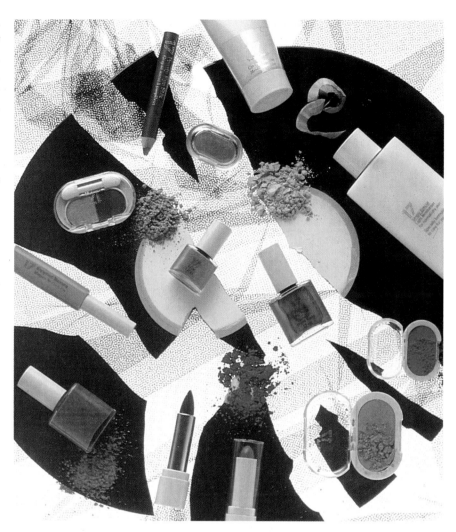

When you start collecting your basic make-up kit, don't be so overawed by the vast range of colours that you end up with 20 eye shadows and no blusher! Picture (above) courtesy of Boots.
A good collection of brushes, like these from Stephen Glass, is another necessity.

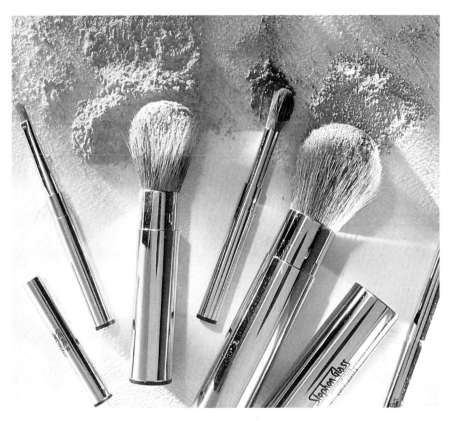

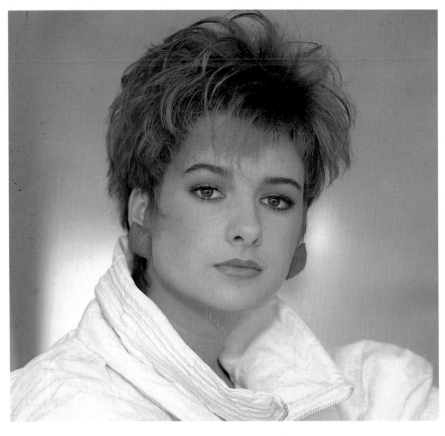

your face changes colour according to the different seasons of the year.

Blushers, one on the pink side, one on the coral, to tone with whatever eye make-up and lipstick you are using.

Translucent face powder, loose, to set your make-up and hold it all together. You might also need a compressed powder to take with you and touch up with during the day.

Eyeshadows, two or three in the same colour range are all you need to begin with to lighten and lift your eyes.

Eyeliner. We all need some form of line around our eyes to open them up and allow the make-up to look complete. This may be a small half line smudged discreetly under the bottom lashes or a line all the way along the lid, close to the top ones.

Mascara, is absolutely essential; even if your lashes are tinted you'll still need a fine coating of mascara to make them noticeable beside your eyeshadows.

Lip pencils. Some people recommend a lip pencil two or three shades darker than your lip colour, but this can create problems. Not only does it mean buying several colours to match your lipsticks, but also, when the lipstick comes off after a few hours, you are left with an unnatural line framing your lips. Opt instead for a more natural colour, which gives the lips definition and helps to stop lipstick from 'bleeding', but doesn't look too false.

Mirrors. Whether you have good or bad eyesight, it's a good idea to have a magnifying mirror as well as an ordinary one. This will help you

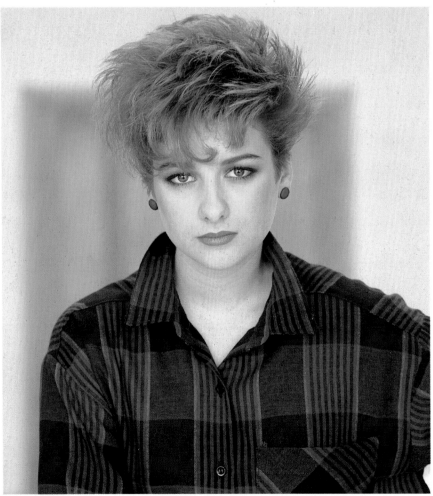

These pictures from the Taylor Ferguson salon in Glasgow show how the same girl can look totally different with a little body added to her hair and a change of make-up colours. It is a good way of making a day to night transformation.

38

check minor details and irritating little faults, like that odd, fine, straggly eyebrow.

Tweezers. Have them at the ready every morning.

A wide hair band or similar, to hold your hair off your face so that it doesn't get covered in make-up but your face does!

Sponges are useful pieces of equipment which do help make-up flow on more easily, though I have my doubts as to whether sponge owners wash them as often as they should, which is every day. To let them sit in the drawer or the make-up bag collecting stale cosmetics and bacteria is courting disaster as far as your face is concerned. If you don't have the time or memory to be scrupulously clean with sponges use the next best and perfectly adequate tool – your fingers, washed.

Brushes. You'll need a nice bushy one, about 5 cm (2 in) wide, for powder, and another, about 4 cm ($1\frac{1}{2}$ in) wide for blusher. Choose a couple of eyeshadow brushes with flat, square ends about 5 mm ($\frac{1}{4}$ in) wide. A good, long lip brush will give you the leverage you need to apply your lipstick properly. A stiff eyebrow brush will help you make the best of these face-framing features, and an old mascara wand is a handy little item for separating lashes, particularly in between coats.

Things to bear in mind

There are a couple of points to remember before beginning. It's a good idea to put on your make-up before you dress for the day, and then apply lipstick last. Once you're proficient at applying cosmetics there shouldn't be any trace of make-up on your clothes, but you don't want to risk ruining them while you're still learning. Confidence is the key to good make-up application. If you apply the minimum amount of each product and you know what your routine is, the chances of you making mistakes will be minimized and you will feel less nervous about putting it all on. It's when you are impatient and edgy that things get knocked over and mistakes and messes are made. The knowledge that what you are about to do is easy will automatically give you the confidence you need, and remember that the same rule applies to make-up as to everything else – practice makes perfect.

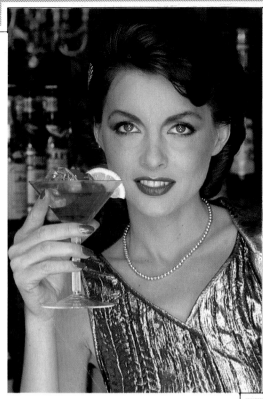

Two examples which show just how different make-up can look. *Right:* A ritzy, sophisticated cocktail look from Almay. *Below:* A young, casual look to suit everyday living from Alan International.

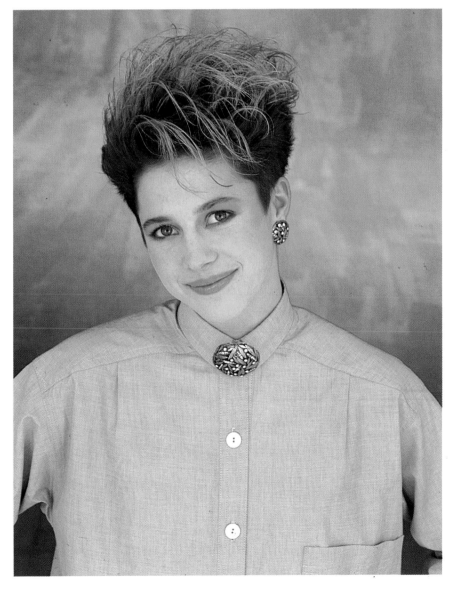

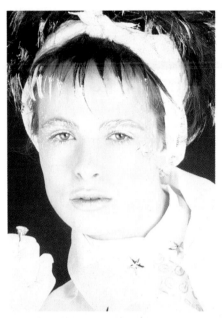

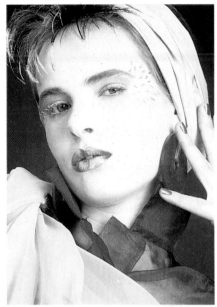

Play with cosmetic colours and match them to your clothes, to one another, even to your moods. Remember that different mediums of make-up: powders, creams, gels, pencils and crayons etc, achieve a different intensity of colour. Don't forget too that to achieve a more vibrant look, perhaps for the evening, you don't necessarily have to apply more of the product. The two pictures on the left, from Boots No 17, reflect soft and pretty pinks and purples while the picture below from Maybelline portrays a delicate blend of pinks and blues. The strong red and black look from Boots No 17 on the right shows to what degree you can go to match your make-up to your clothes.

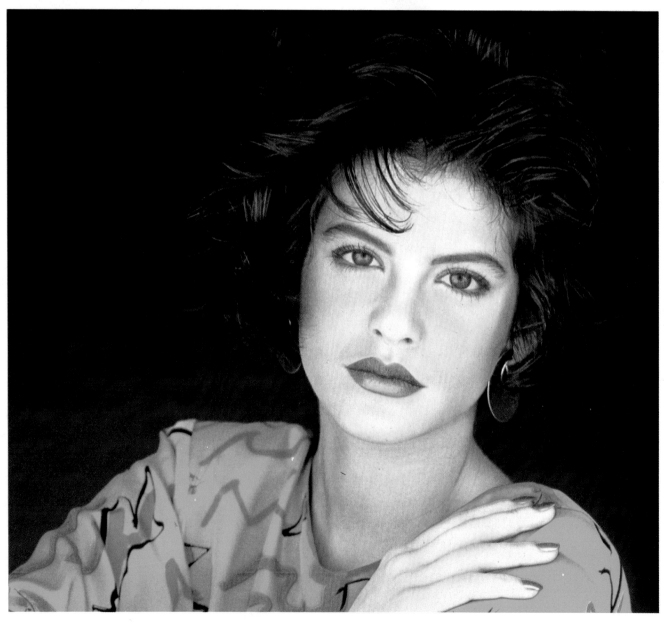

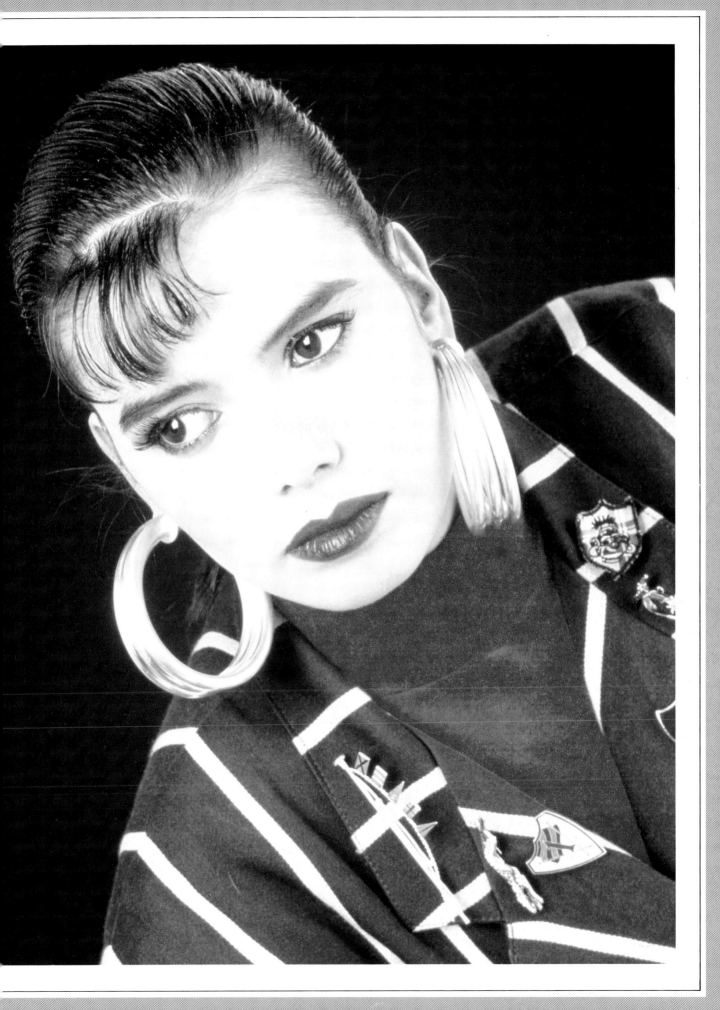

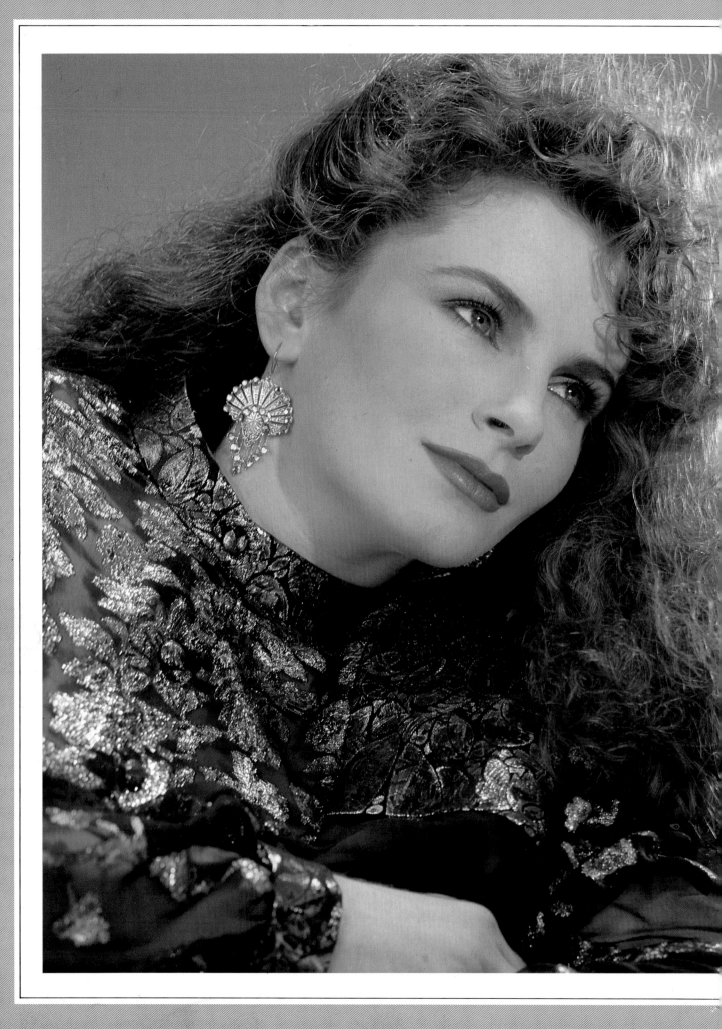

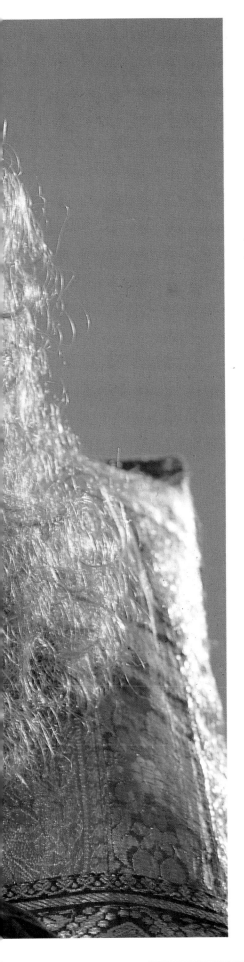

Laying the foundation

To get the very best out of your foundation, you will have to have completed your morning skin-care routine, which probably includes toning and, if your skin needs it, moisturizing. Moisturizer will help the skin maintain adequate moisture levels, to keep it looking smooth and supple. A well-chosen base of moisture will prolong the lasting properties of your foundation and help to prevent colour change from occurring. It may be, though, that your skin is so oily it doesn't need moisturizer, just a fine spray of water to 'seal' the make-up and help guard against the dehydrating effects of the day ahead.

Choosing the right colour

If your face is naturally highly coloured, perhaps with exceptionally ruddy cheeks or with a tendency to redden down the centre panel, it may be that you need to apply corrective colour before your foundation. A green foundation under your normal one will cover up any unsightly redness, and, if you then use a foundation with as much beige as your natural skin tone allows, this will also help to counteract the

Your foundation should never appear noticeable as though you're trying to disguise your face. It should be there to enhance the natural skin colour. This warm look was achieved using Almay's Silk and Spice Collection.

problem, as beiges do contain small amounts of green. The darker your basic skin tone, the more colour 'lifting' will be required, and sallow complexions can benefit from the use of pink-toned foundations.

If you don't like the idea of using two foundations on your face (the colour corrective ones are very light, so there should be no question of heaviness), some companies actually do pre-make-up colour washes. If you've got a problem with blemishes, then hunt for a cover stick which exactly matches your foundation – a tone lighter or darker will magnify your problem, not conceal it – and apply it after your foundation. Or, alternatively, opt for a medicated foundation, which will help heal and dry the skin, camouflage it effectively and at the same time give excellent coverage.

The aim of foundation is to be protective and to give a natural, even skin tone, not to make you look as though you are about to go to a masked ball! The most common mistakes people make with make-up involves the real basics, foundation and blusher, and it is all too easy to use the wrong foundation time and time again, especially as they all seem so wonderful. To get exactly the right product you must know your skin type and be able to analyze your natural colouring. Study your face closely and see whether you can detect a tendency towards a natural pinkness or beigeness. The skin just above the wrist or on the inside of the arm is pretty much the same shade as on the face so have a double check in these areas if you are in any doubt. Since you want to achieve a natural look and enhance your skin rather than disguise it, choose a tone no more than one shade lighter or darker than the natural one, and always check the colour of the foundation on your skin in natural light before you buy.

What kind of skin?

Another thing which might help you select the colour of your foundation is knowledge of its pH content. (The term pH means potential of hydrogen, and is a rating of acidity or alkalinity on a scale of 0–14.) The pH of skin ranges from 4.5 to 5.5, but cleansing and toning agents, like shampoo and conditioning products on hair, can alter this value. Cleansing with soap and water, for instance, can change it to about 7. If skin has a pH of more than 7.1, the foundation tends to stand out from the natural skin tone and if you find this to be the case, select a colour one tone lighter than your natural skin tone. If, however, your skin is acid, foundations will have a tendency to be absorbed into the face and disappear, in which case plump for a make-up one tone darker than your own. You will soon known if your foundation doesn't suit. Your complexion will be either shiny or dry and parched-looking, any irregularities will appear emphasized

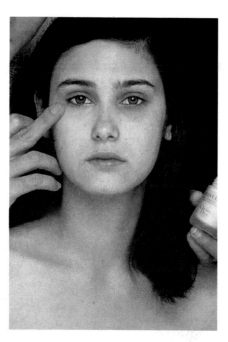

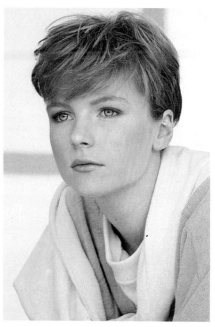

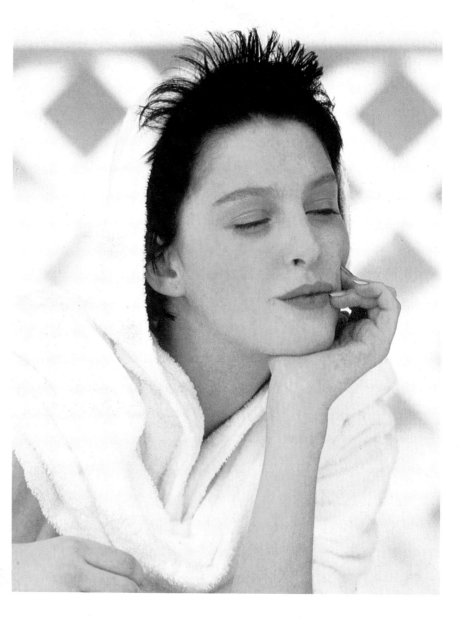

Getting the correct colour of foundation is crucial. Test the product on the inside of the wrist or arm and choose a tone that is no more than one shade lighter or darker than your natural one. Picture, top left, courtesy of Dior, illustrates a dusky, olive complexion while the photograph top right, from Almay, shows a much fairer skin. Main picture, this page, shows the fresh, natural look. Courtesy of Boots No 7.
Opposite: Mary Quant Cosmetics created this bronze-faced beauty/party look.

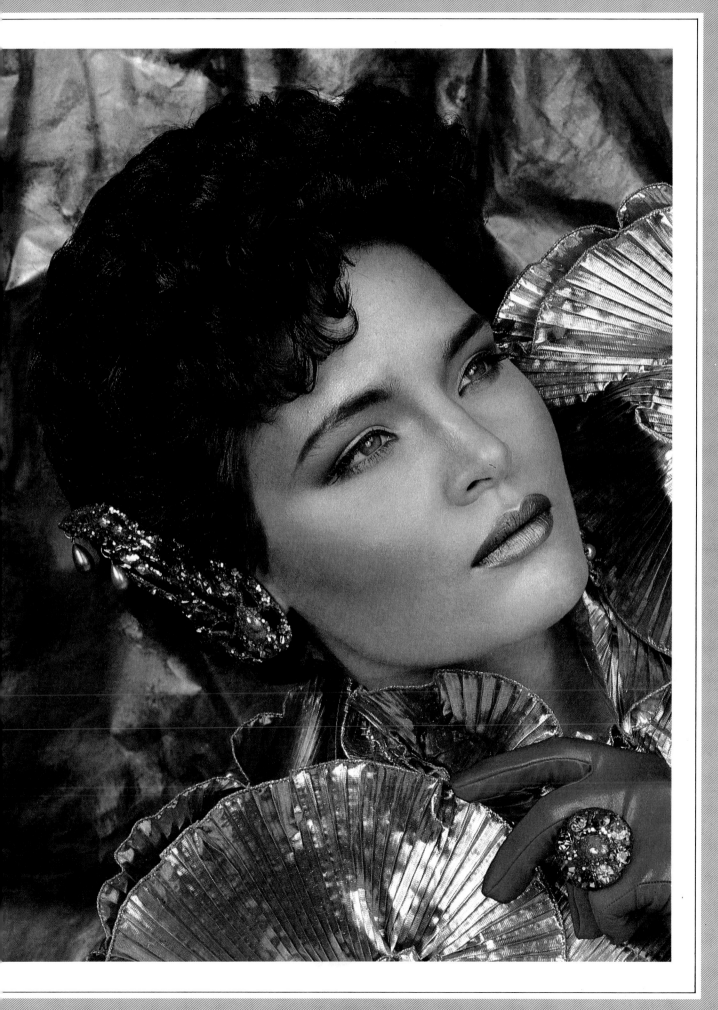

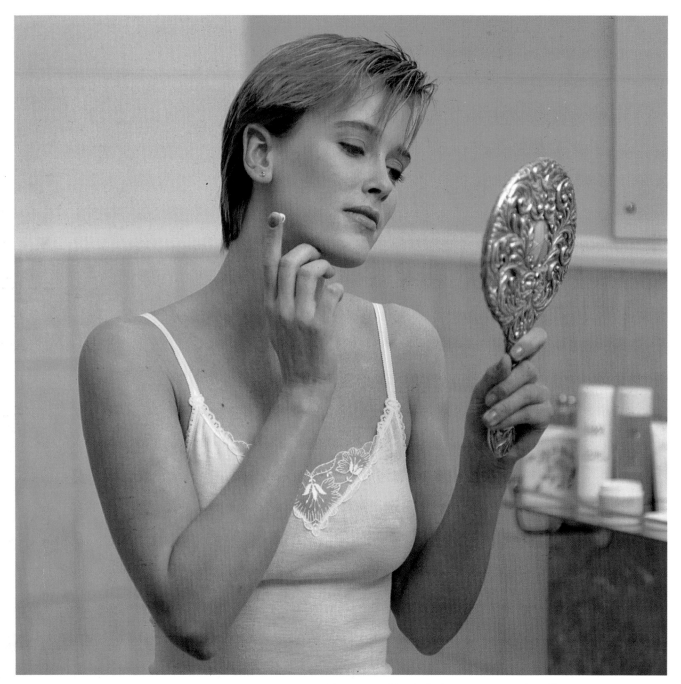

Work in your foundation with quick, light movements and be sure to blend all the areas in together. Fingers are easier to use than sponges and are more than adequate as long as they are scrupulously clean. Photograph courtesy of Almay.

rather than smoothed down, and there will be definite areas of colour change.

Obviously the drier your complexion, the more creamy your foundation will need to be. If you have oily skin, you want to look for an oil-free make-up and, if you have combination skin, you may need two foundations to do the job properly. If you have badly blemished skin you should be thinking about a medicated make-up, and if your skin seems particularly allergic or sensitive, then choose from one of the many hypo-allergic products on the market.

Applying foundation

When putting on your foundation, make sure that your hands are clean and apply the cosmetic either directly from the container or first blobbed on to the palm of your hand. Work with quick, light movements, dabbing the foundation on your face in dots a short distance apart and working on one section at a time. Blend the areas gently into one another. If you prefer to use a sponge rather than your fingers, it must always be damp and must be kept very clean indeed. Sponges make for a nice, even coverage and, slightly dampened, are very easy to use.

Another tip on cleanliness here is never to let anyone else – not even Mum – use your own foundation. Germs can spread so very easily, and months of good skin care can be wasted in one thoughtless moment. Remember, too, that if you are using a water-based foundation, you really have to get your skates on. This dries almost as soon as it is applied to the skin, so don't stop for a chat or a cup of coffee when you are working it in. It's a good idea to start at the forehead and work down – over the temples to the eyelids, cheeks, jaw line and chin, shading away until you reach the throat. If you have particularly red earlobes covering them with a dot of foundation can't do any harm, but there really is no need to work foundation into the throat. Your make-up base should match your neck, making it unnecessary to cover it. Foundation on the neck will not only show up any wrinkles you might have, but will also come off on the clothes you are wearing and make a mess.

A little foundation dotted on the eyelids does help eye make-up to stay fast as well as evening out the skin tone, but you may prefer to choose one of the corrective make-ups specially formulated for those more delicate areas. In any case, be sure not to plaster your eyebrows with the product, as they will clog up and look unnatural. If there are blue veins on your lids you may need a slightly heavier foundation than you are using on the rest of your face. If you have wrinkles around the eyes – and most of us do from quite an early age – then tread very gently when applying foundation to this area. Pat, rather than stroke, it on so the skin won't be pulled, and don't pile on too much. An even better idea is to use a thinner, filmier foundation than your normal one. A lighter foundation than usual, patted on gently and well blended, will help correct problem areas like dark circles and bags under the eyes, lines around the

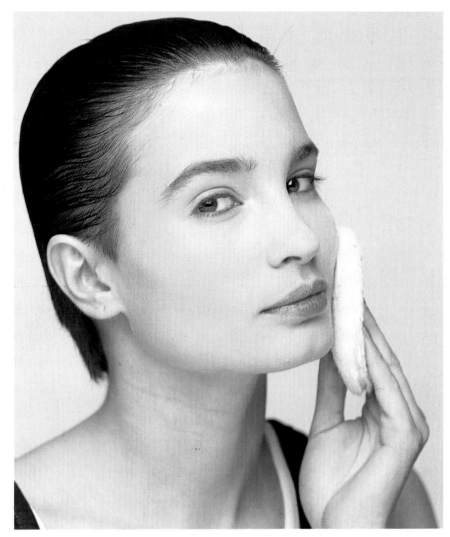

One good application of loose powder in the morning, with an occasional touch up with compressed powder during the day, will preserve your make-up and give it that finished look. Picture courtesy of Mary Quant Cosmetics.

nose and mouth, and crows' feet. Now study yourself in the mirror and look for any areas which might come to an abrupt end rather than mingle in with the next, and correct them by blending the foundation further.

Powder

The finishing touch to your base is your powder. The same rule about enhancement rather than exaggeration applies here also. Powder shouldn't paint your face, but allow what you've already done to show through, preserving and sealing your foundation in the process. Most of today's powders are translucent, light and only

slightly tinted. One good application of loose powder in the morning, touched up occasionally with compressed powder during the day, should be enough to see you through until the evening. As with any other product, keep the amount used over wrinkled areas down to a minimum, otherwise you will only make them more conspicuous. Take a clean piece of cotton wool and gently but firmly pat the powder wherever you have applied make-up. Remove the excess powder by flicking over these areas with a large, soft brush in the direction the hair grows. Now you have laid the foundation and are ready to make your face really come alive by careful shaping and shading.

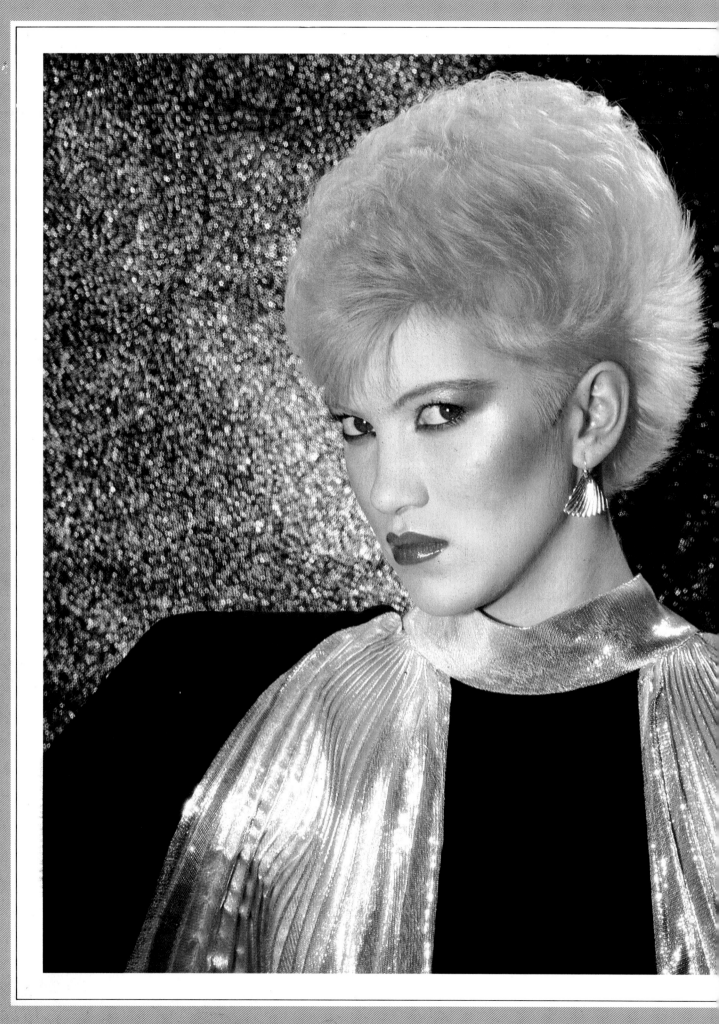

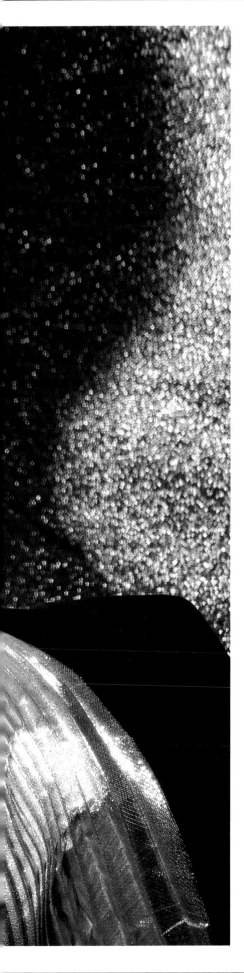

Face shaping

Before you go on to learn how make-up can best flatter your looks, it's important to study your face and get to know its shape, as well as that of your eyes and nose, so that you can apply your cosmetics accordingly. A perfectly proportioned face is one that has equal measurements from the tip of the nose to the lowest part of the chin and from the outer corner of the eye to the tip of the nose. Facial features and expressions are determined by the bony structures supporting the muscles and the fat over these muscles. There are particular ways of applying make-up to enhance or play down certain face shapes, but sometimes the rules need to be disregarded or broken, for instance, don't concentrate too rigidly on applying make-up to elongate a square face if it doesn't make the most of your eyes. The key is to get to know the guidelines and adapt them to suit yourself – you may even discover a few tips of your own!

Changing shapes

A round face is often chubby, and its features need to be sharpened to create an overall illusion of slimness, especially around the chin and jaws. This type of face shape would benefit from two foundations, a fairly dark shade on the outer areas of the face and a lighter one down the centre panel.

An oval face is considered by many to be the most perfectly proportioned, although sometimes this shape can exaggerate its own good lines. The forehead, for instance, may be too broad for the rest of the face, and there may be too great a gap between the eyebrows and the hairline. The distance between the bottom lip and chin may also be too long. Good eyes and a soft hairstyle will draw attention away from the high forehead and a good, well made-up mouth will counteract the length between the lower lip and the chin. Highlighter blended into the chin area will help make the best of this face shape and divert attention from what might be too broad a forehead.

A heart-shaped face is small and delicate, broad at the temples and narrow at the chin, and you'll have to make certain that you strike a good balance between these two areas.

A square face is usually large with strong features. The width at the temples and jaw and height from the hairline to the bottom of the chin are all about the same. This gives a general impression of too much width and too little height, which needs to be balanced by shading and blushing so that the one does not dominate the other. Blusher at the temples, careful shading from cheek to jaw and a little highlighter on the chin all help to achieve this.

A triangular face is one with either very broad temples and a sharply pointed chin or a narrow forehead

The flick of a blusher brush can make all the difference to the contours of a face. Greater depth of colour, as pictured on this model from a collection of photographs from Alan International, is often needed for the evening.

and broad chin. If you have broad temples, then you need to shade them to make them appear less broad, and shade the chin to shorten it. If you have a narrow forehead and broad chin you'll need to narrow the sides of the jaw by shading and broaden the temples with blusher.

An oblong face can either be a long version of a square face or an angular version of an oval one. It often has high cheekbones and wide areas between the eyes and

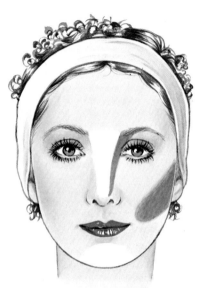

The chubbiness of a round face needs to be sharpened to create an overall illusion of slimness.

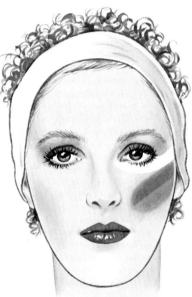

An oval face is thought to be the ideal shape on which to work, although sometimes the forehead can be proportionately too broad.

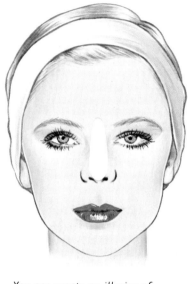

You can create an illusion of length to a short nose like this one by adding a slight touch of highlighter from the bridge all the way down to the tip.

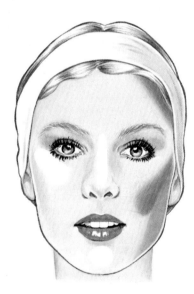

This is a square face with large, strong features which can give an impression of too much width and too little height. Careful blending and shading is needed here to ensure that one feature does not dominate another.

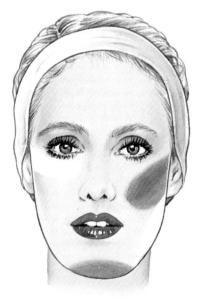

An oblong face often has high cheekbones and a wide area between the eyes and brows. Play up the eyes and soften any harsh angles.

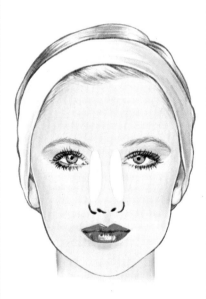

A long nose can be shortened by applying highlighter at the side and shader on the tip.

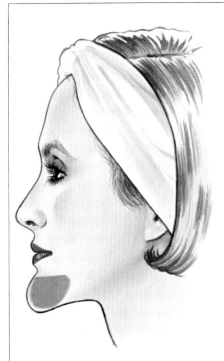

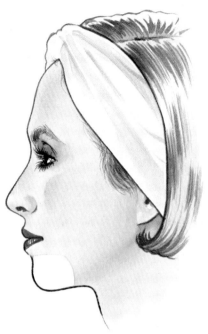

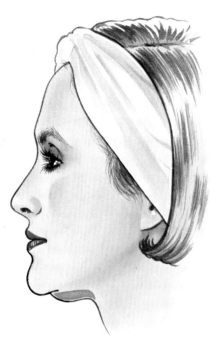

Shader can be used to minimize a protruding chin although when a correction as large as this one needs to be made, try using loose powder a shade darker than your normal one.

By highlighting what you are proud of and shading what you want to minimize you can accentuate your best features and disguise those you are not too proud of.

You can even shade underneath a sagging double chin perhaps with foundation one tone darker than your normal one, to make it less noticeable.

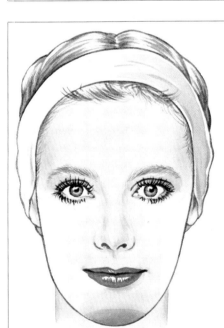

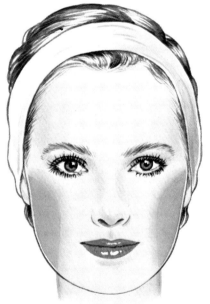

You can add width to a narrow jawline by just lightening it.

A broad jawline can be subtly shaded to give it an illusion of slimness.

brows. Here you'll want to play up the eyes and mouth and soften any harsh angles at the temples with shader. Decrease the illusion of length by applying shader across the chin, and highlight the brow-bones.

Improving on nature

There are other corrective tricks which can be worked with deft use of the brush, blusher and shader, but remember, that any corrective make-up must be done with subtlety. To correct a protruding chin apply shadow to the areas to be played down. Conversely, if your chin recedes, lighten in a shallow area. Play down a sagging double chin by applying a foundation one tone darker than your normal one on the problem area. To create an illusion of length to a short nose add a delicate touch of highlighter from the bridge all the way down to the tip. A protruding nose can

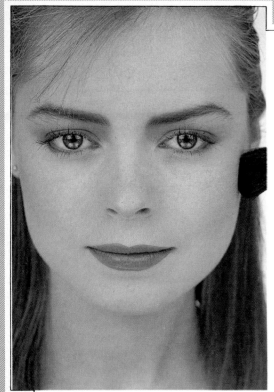

Blusher comes in a wide range of shades. For best results, as this picture above from Almay shows, they should be blended well in with a brush. Take colour right up to the temple to really brighten the face. Picture, right, courtesy of L'Oreal.

be made to appear less so with highlighter at the sides and shader on the tip. You can lighten a narrow jaw line to give it width, and play down a broad one with shadow. The rule to remember is that you highlight something you are proud of and want to draw attention to but shade what you want to minimize. You can accentuate good bones with light make-up, yet draw attention away from a feature you're none too proud of – perhaps a broad nose or a double chin – with a dark one.

Blusher and highlighter

Blusher adds colour, vitality and 'life' to the face, whereas highlighter adds width, not necessarily accentuating as it does so. Continuously blend and smudge to achieve the most subtle of effects. Use loose powder a shade darker than your normal one for the most discreet of results. Any over-drastic corrections will look hideous by daylight and emphasize the very feature you have painstakingly tried to disguise.

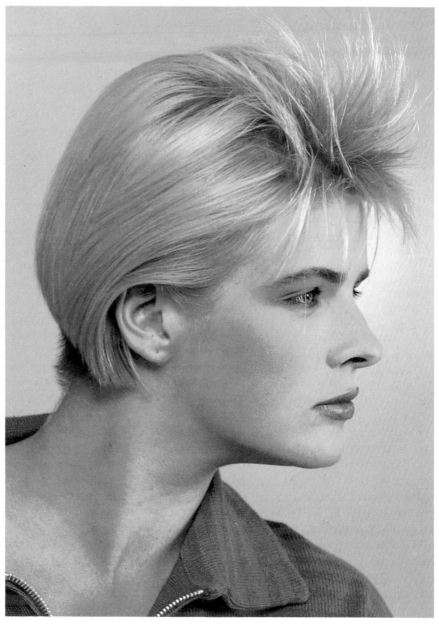

Blushers, shaders and highlighters come in many forms, and blushers are available in all colours, from pink through to bright red and from russet brown through to yellow. Shaders and highlighters range from very white, pearlized products, to darkest brown. Shaping and blushing can be done either after applying foundation or after applying powder, depending on the types of products you are using (gel, powder, cream, etc), but the general rule is that powder should be applied on powder, cream on cream. So if you are using a powder blusher, apply it after your loose powder. A cream blusher, on the other hand, should be applied before powder but after foundation. One good professional tip, however, totally breaks this rule but works a treat. If your skin type permits, apply a gel or cream blusher underneath your powder and a powder blusher in the same colour on top. This will ensure that your rosy glow will last well into the night.

Right: A beautifully co-ordinated make-up from Almay which illustrates how an outfit of clothes, and cosmetics like eye shadow, shader and lipstick can all co-ordinate with one another.

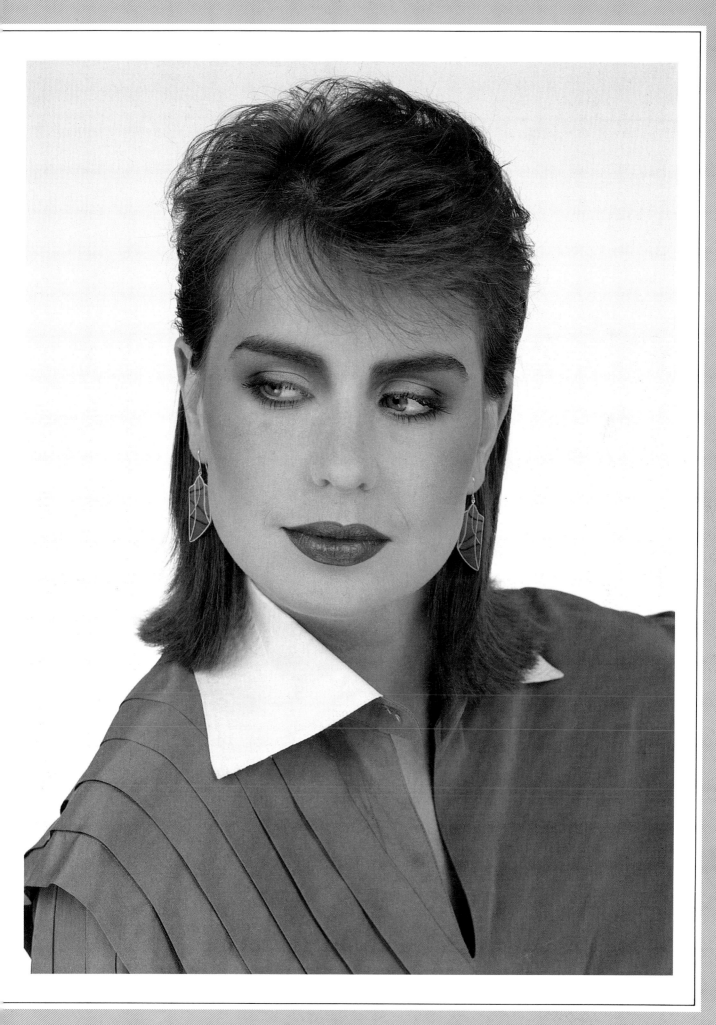

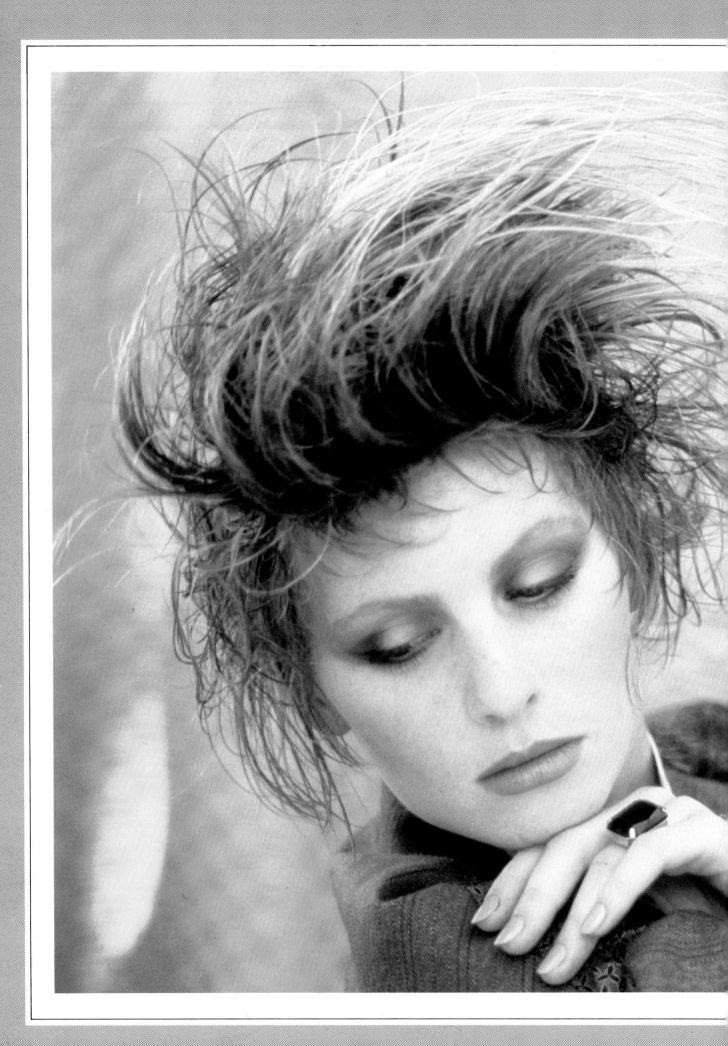

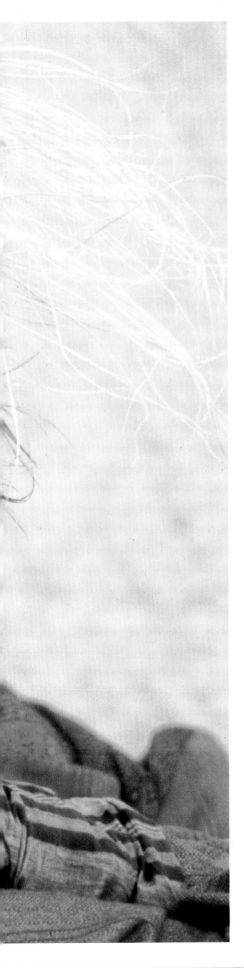

Eyes right

Eyes are where the fun really begins. More than any of your other facial features, your eyes give you an opportunity to play around with make-up, to experiment with colours and designs which make the very best of these 'windows of your soul'. Don't forget that your eyes are not only your means of looking out at the world, they are also an important means of communicating with others. They are the focal point of your face and the true expression of your mood and personality.

I recommend that while you are experimenting with eye make-up you do so at the weekend when you don't have to go to work the next day. You should never drag the skin around the eyes or put it under too much pressure, as eyes are sensitive and you don't want to turn up at work looking like a red-eyed rabbit. For the same reason don't try to experiment with too many colours and designs at once, no matter how much you may be itching to get to grips with that new eye shadow palette. Instead, try out one new look a week until you get the perfect colour 'wardrobe'.

What type of eye make-up?

There is a baffling choice of eye make-up types and colours avail-

You can have more fun with eye make-up than with cosmetics on any other part of your face as there are such a myriad of colours, and make-up mediums, to choose from. This look was created by Boots No 7.

able. Creams, liquids, compact powders, powder cream, sticks and transparent tints all add to the vast range of eye shadows on the market. Cream shadows are easy to apply, but it is hard to control the density of colour, and they do crease easily. Pencils are useful little items, as you can direct the colour exactly where you want it whilst still avoiding sharp lines – smudging is the key with all make-up. Pencils are available in two forms. There are thin ones, which are good for directing colour on small, delicate areas, or there are chubbier ones. They tend to go blunt easily, so you'll need sharpeners, but do make sure that these are used only for your eye pencils. Keep well away from younger brothers and sisters who might borrow them for their crayons!

Powder shadows create a far softer effect than pencils, and have a greater flexibility of application. They can be put on straight from the palette with a sponge applicator (usually provided by the manufacturer, although you will still need some good ones of your own) or wet, with a long-handled brush for balance and control. When using water and a brush – and this method will not only intensify colour but ensure that the eye make-up stays on – simply dip the brush into a pot of water and then stroke it once or twice along your darkest eye shadow colour. If you paint a little on to the back of your hand at this stage, it should stay smoothly where it is and not come off in streaks. Remember that it is much easier to add more colour than to take it away if you've put on too much, so

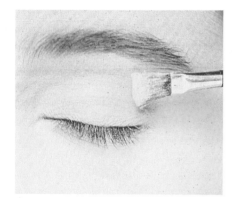

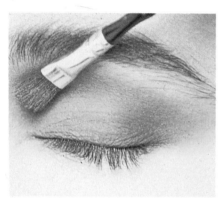

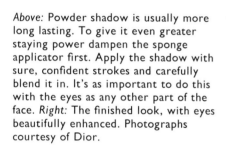

Above: Powder shadow is usually more long lasting. To give it even greater staying power dampen the sponge applicator first. Apply the shadow with sure, confident strokes and carefully blend it in. It's as important to do this with the eyes as any other part of the face. *Right:* The finished look, with eyes beautifully enhanced. Photographs courtesy of Dior.

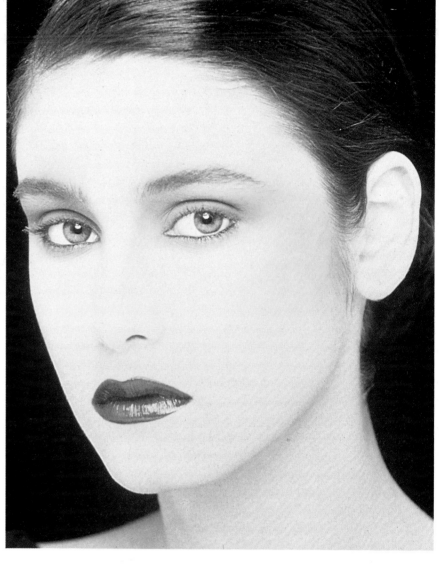

go cautiously. If you only have one brush, rinse it and wipe it with a tissue before going on to a lighter colour. Obviously what you do with your make-up will depend on the shape, size and setting of your eyes, but as a general rule the stronger shades go on the lids, while lighter tones are blended outward to near the brow bone, where highlighter is applied.

What colours?

There is no more bewildering make-up advice in magazines than that on eye make-up. Colours change from season to season to suit fashion moods. One month it's drama, the next it's pastel hues, and we are constantly being told to be adventurous and change our eye make-up. Drama is all very well for those who look or feel dramatic, or enjoy experimenting, but most of us know which colours suit us best, and I can't blame anyone for sticking to them. After all, if you've got brilliant blue eyes, are you really going to want to detract from them by wearing green eye shadow just because jade green is the fashion colour of the month? But it doesn't necessarily follow, of course, that blue eye shadow should be worn by people with blue eyes and grey by those with grey eyes — there are a myriad of colours and shades in between that you can choose from.

The best way of deciding which eye colours suit you is to use them and take a long, hard look in the mirror. Does the end result actually do anything for you? Does it make your eyes look 'alive', or flatter your hair colour or complexion? If not, then think again. As a general guideline — and this is very general as I'm a great believer in rules being made to be broken where beauty is concerned — if you have brown eyes and dark hair and skin try a combination of silver grey and heather pink shadows.

There is, of course, absolutely no reason why you shouldn't be outrageous sometimes — for a special occasion perhaps or even a fancy dress. Miners have illustrated the true meaning of face painting in this photograph.

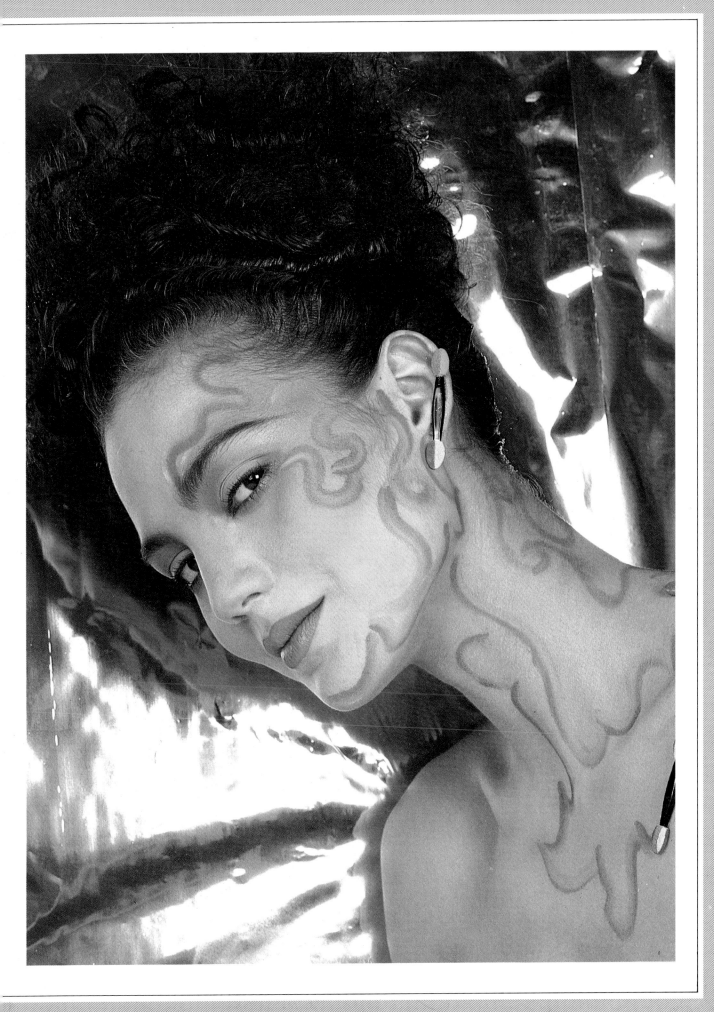

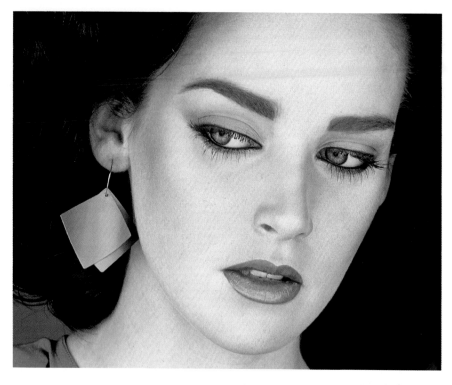

This can be very flattering against a dark, olive skin. Be careful with pink and purple eye shadows, though, as not everyone can wear them. On some of us pink shadow simply makes us look as though we've had a bad night! If you have hazel or green eyes, an auburn complexion and creamy skin, try combinations of grey, green and gold shadows. Peach and brown tones are flattering for those of us with grey-blue eyes, brown hair and pale skin, while green-blue and gold-brown are nice combinations for all those blue-eyed, golden-haired blondes there are amongst us.

Making the most of your eyes

Very few of us have what are considered to be 'normal' eyes — well-set, well-shaped and in good proportion to the rest of the face. If you have eyes like this, then almost anything goes as far as eye make-up is concerned, but for the rest of us, there are a few tricks which help make the most of eyes, no matter what their faults are.

Small eyes need enlarging, so be generous with the highlighter. You want to open up the eye, so avoid any sharp, dark lines, and instead try to achieve a three-dimensional effect. Start with a colour scheme of, for example, white or very pale blue, violet and dove grey. Colour the entire lid with your brightest, softest tone, in this case white, for the enlarging effect. Now blend in a little violet on the centre of the lid to accentuate this area. Then apply a soft sweep of your deepest colour, grey, along the brow line, but not

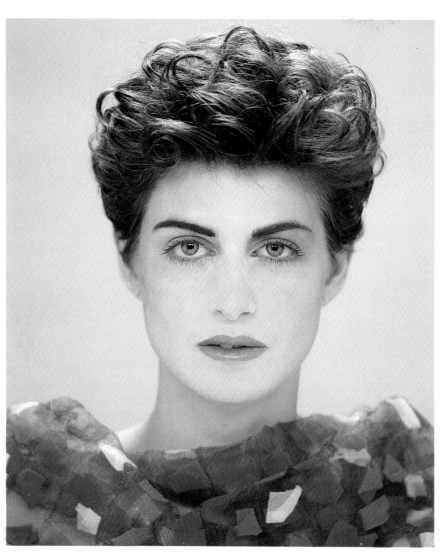

Top left: Blue eye shadow can look stunning on certain people but doesn't suit all of us. Picture courtesy of Maybelline. *Bottom left:* Make-up can match the focal point of an outfit, in this case a scarf. Picture courtesy of Perfect Colour by Cutex.

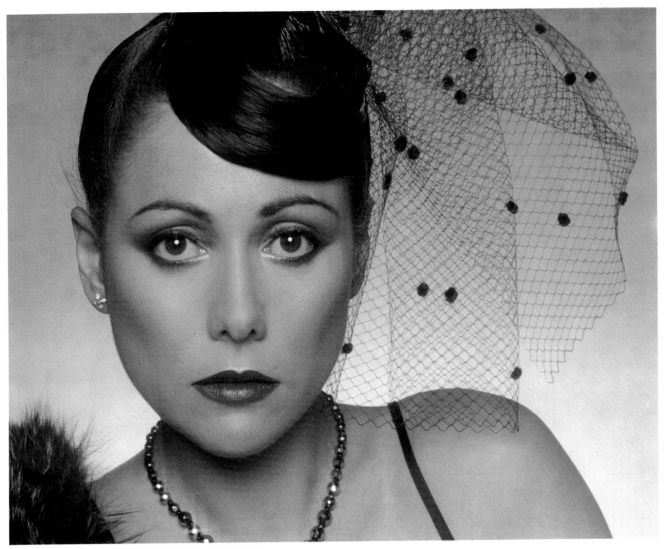

Large, round eyes are too good a feature to be played down, but if they are overemphasized they dominate the face. Greys are ideal smoky colours for this eye shape and here Crimpers have struck a perfect balance.

right up to the eyebrow. You can feel your brow bone protruding between your lid and eyebrow, and your darkest colour should go no further than this. Remember to smudge and blend everything in well together. Smudge in a little of your darkest colour under the bottom lashes, and concentrate your mascara, with fine, sweeping strokes, on the other lashes.

Owners of large eyes are lucky people, as they can so often get away with no eye shadow at all, just lashings of mascara or, if their lashes are tinted or naturally dark and lustrous, nothing! Large eyes can be a problem, though, if they dominate the face to such an extent that every other feature pales into insignificance. In this

case try and subdue your eyes with dark, subtle colours and blend in a soft, smoky edge of colour near the lashes.

Protruding and heavy-lidded eyes seem large and bulging. Keep well away from anything too bright or frosted, as this will only make your eyes appear more prominent. You want a more subdued effect, with darker shadows close to the lashes. If your eyes are also small you can make an exception here and place just a touch of highlighter at the inner corners of the eyes to open them up. Try blending a sombre but rich colour on the upper lid of the eye. Plum is a good, smouldering shade, and then apply a matching tone — in this case pink would be ideal —

along the brow bone area and perhaps under the lower lashes. This will help to illuminate the upper part of the eye and take away the interest from the protruding lids.

Deep-set eyes can look rather stern, with prominent brow bones. You want to soften their effect and bring them forward with pale, light colours. Take a pale colour like yellow and blend it into the entire area from the lashes to the brow bone. Now take a cream and shade in along the brow bone, winging it out along the crease. Finally, take a gold or light bronze pearlized colour and blend it into the area underneath the arch of the brow and on the centre of the lid.

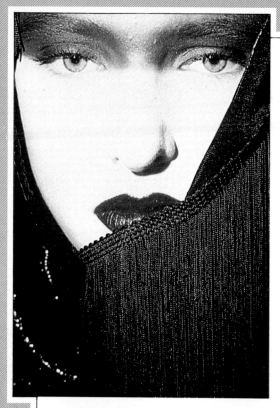

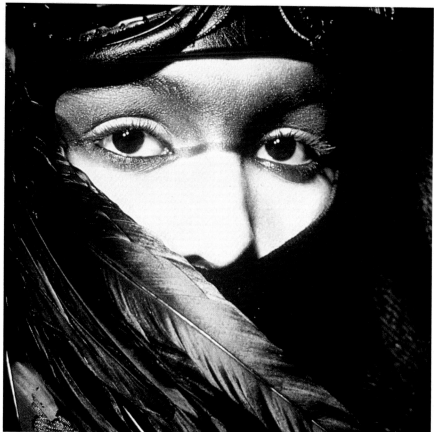

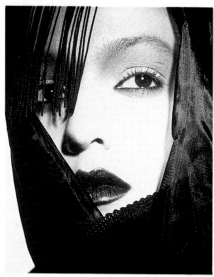

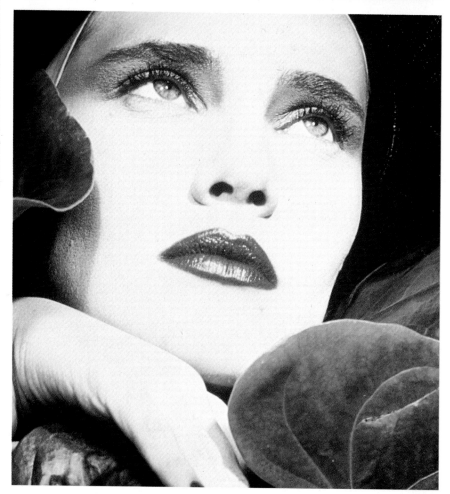

This selection of rainbow colours from Dior not only illustrates the delightful choice of eye shadows available but also what can be done with them. You won't always want to look this dramatic though, and you've really got to be confident of your ability before you try creating anything like these pictures here — otherwise it will just not work. And what a waste of a good product! People should compliment you on how pretty your eyes look, not on your eye shadow colour. So take a long hard look in the mirror and decide whether a shadow really does anything for you before you step out into the streets.

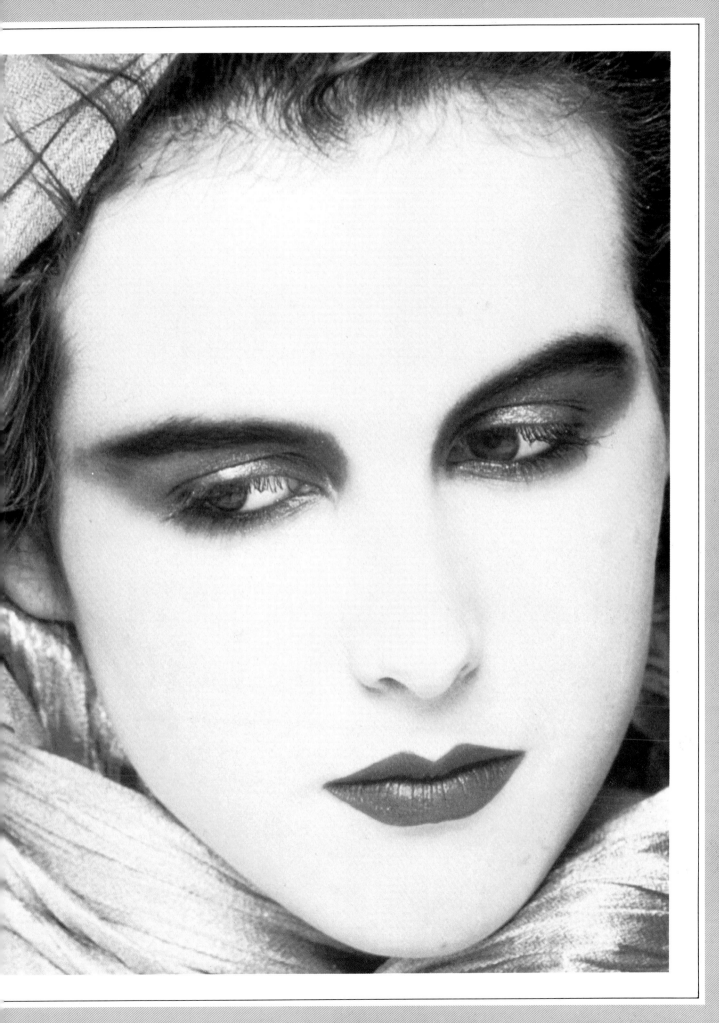

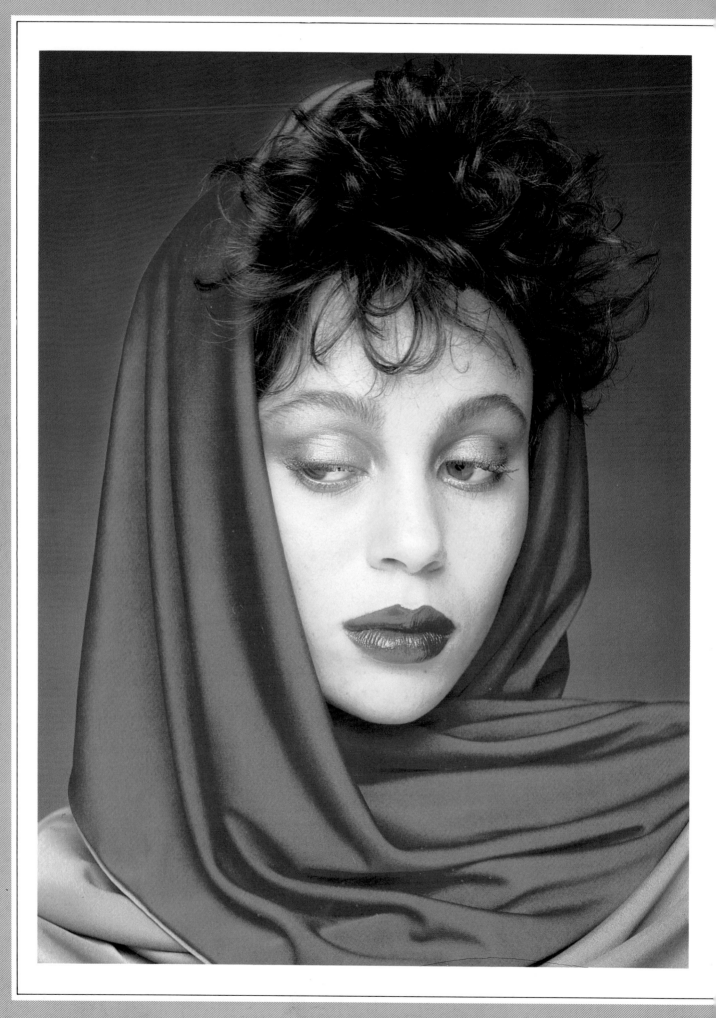

Round eyes can give the face a 'startled' look, so here you need to add height and reduce width. Try highlighting the entire upper lid with a pale tone, like ivory. To contrast, take a dark gold and apply it in the socket line to form a sweeping curve. A very fine line of gold or brown shadow can then be applied close to the upper lashes. Highlight the arch of the brow with a white or cream shadow and then apply a cream or gold shade at the outer corner of the eye.

Heavy lidded eyes are usually large so subdue them with darker shadows close to the lashes. Picture courtesy of Christine at Mane Line.

Almond eyes appear to slant slightly. They are long and narrow with an upward tilt on the outer corners. To overcome this (and you may not want to, as this eye shape can be very attractive), apply dark shadow quite heavily on the lids, at the outer corners and under the bottom lashes. If they are also wide apart, try blending a little dark shadow on the inner corners of the eye near the nose in an upwards direction.

Your eyes are close-set if you have only a small space across the bridge of your nose between your eyes, and you do need to create an illusion of space between them.

Cover over the entire area, from lid to brow bone, with a pale, soft shadow, perhaps an avocado green. Now take a brown or dark green and blend it into the crease and up to the brow bone, creating a wide curve as you move towards the outside of the eye, with a light, moss green highlight underneath the arch of the brow.

If your eyes are wide apart, concentrate your darkest shadows on the inner corners of the eye, and blend the lighter tones of shadow towards the outside. Using this method will help decrease the noticeable width across the bridge of the nose.

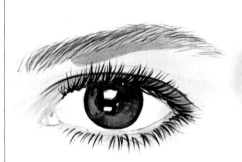

Deep set eyes can be brought forward with the use of pale, irridescent colours blended in an oval around the upper and lower lids.

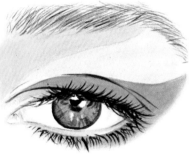

Overhanging lids can be subtly shaded to diminish their prominence with a matt eye shadow which is fairly deep toned.

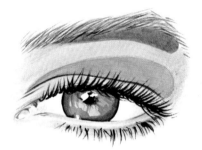

For close-set eyes, bring the area above the eye more forward with a pale shadow and then use a colour to highlight the browbone area.

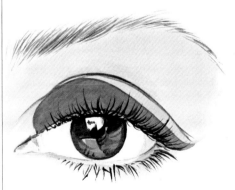

Sombre but rich shadows applied to the upper lids can help bring out heavy-lidded eyes, as does shading the browbone area.

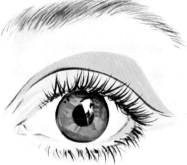

For round eyes, highlight the entire area of the upper lid, blend a sweeping curve of colour into the socket and add a fine bright line near to the lashes.

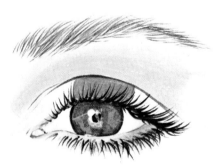

Enlarge small eyes by covering the entire lid with a bright, soft colour and accentuate the centre lid area with a more definite but contrasting shade.

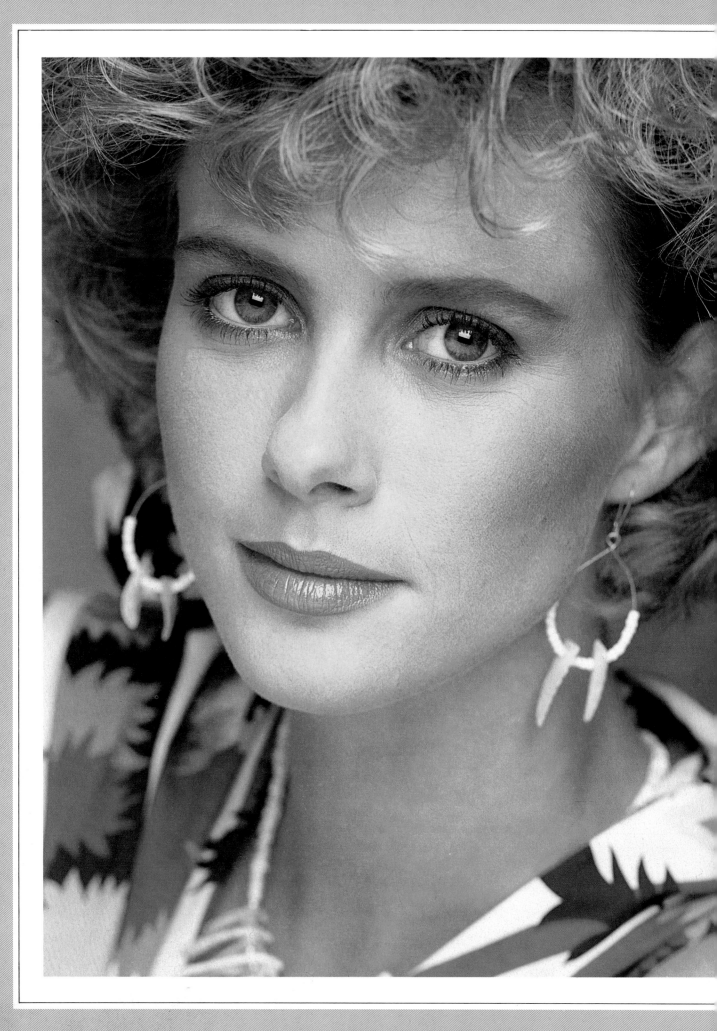

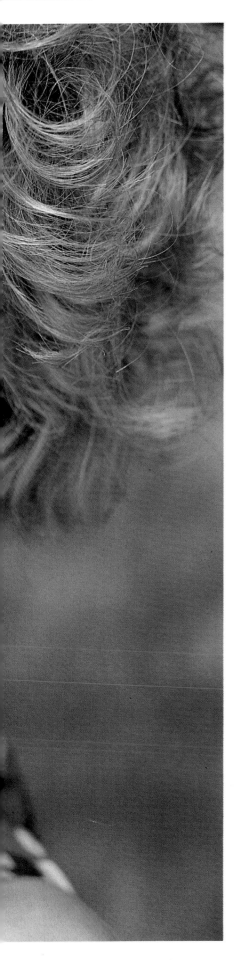

Setting the sights

Well-made-up eyes don't just stop at shadow. There are many other products which can be applied to eyes to frame them and provide them with the extra definition and emphasis they may need, in addition to giving a finished look to those expertly applied colours!

Eyeliner

Eyeliner, although used far less in recent years, still plays an important part in the whole process of eye make-up. The main point to remember is to keep it discreet. The days of naked eyes surrounded by thick, dark liner are long gone. Liner should be used as a tool to emphasize the lashes, not to make a positive statement on its own. If your make-up is stronger than the quality of your eyes then you have too much on. People should say to you 'don't your eyes look pretty today', not 'what unusual make-up'.

Clever use of liner can open, lengthen or emphasize the eye, depending on how it is used. If used too obviously, it will serve no purpose other than to date your make-up. The line should be fine and soft, applied with a tapered brush close to the roots of the lashes – not beyond them. Some-

Although eye shadow plays a prominent role in the making up of eyes, it is by no means the only one. Eye liner and mascara have an equally important part to play as Max Factor have demonstrated here with products from their Outdoor Girl Range.

times a coloured shadow can do the job nicely. To stop the effect looking top-heavy, carefully apply a fragmented line close to the eye underneath the lower lashes.

You can also use kohl to accentuate the eyes if you use strong make-up tones and have the confidence to carry it off. This is a soft eye make-up, available in different colours in pencil form, similar to that used by Indian women. It should be applied near the top lashes and inner rim of the eye and cleverly smudged in to create the softly smouldering and romantic effect associated with it. If you wear contact lenses, however, don't use any make-up product on the inner rim of the eye, as you risk it drying and breaking off into the eye, causing unnecessary discomfort.

Eyebrows and eyelashes

Eyebrows

Eyebrow pencils are sometimes useful if you have a particularly fair colouring, but never go for anything harsh; a grey or brown should be strong enough to give the necessary definition. Don't rely on eyebrow pencils to shape your brows and use them as an excuse to pluck away mercilessly. It's far more attractive, and more natural, to have thick, well-shaped brows which are all your very own. If you are using a pencil, apply it with short, light strokes

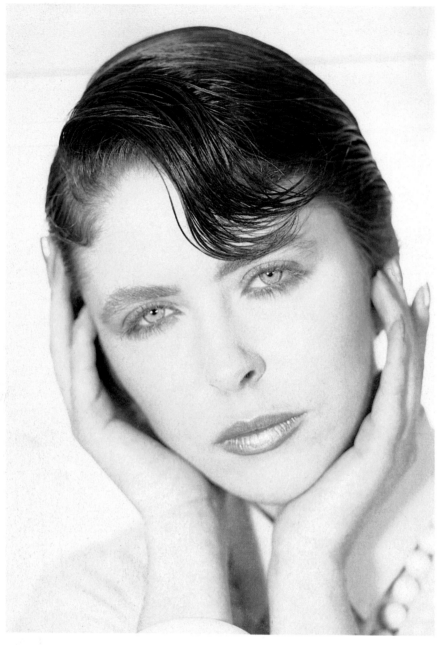

By all means use a little pencil to emphasize brows, but do so with soft, feathery strokes as shown in this picture by John Dacosta. Here he has matched up the look with the use of a soft brown mascara.

and use it to enhance the natural shape of the eye, particularly where the brow might be a bit sparse. If you allow your pencil to become a little bit blunt it will help prevent any harsh lines. A sweeping eyebrow is usually the most attractive as it frees a lot of eye area for make-up and gives width to the face. Moreover, it not only opens up the eyes but gives interest to a narrow face, and can help balance a large mouth or nose. Another natural brow shape

is a rounded one, which follows the contour of the frontal bone and tapers at the end, taking in the round shape of the eye. This best suits large eyes and very wide foreheads. A more angular-shaped brow can give interest to a round face and can be exploited to give it contour and elegance.

Eyelashes

An eyelash curler may look like a weapon of torture, but it provides an easy way of giving lashes lift and sweeping them high. If you do use one, curl the lashes before you put on mascara, and gently squeeze to lift the lashes. Don't re-curl after you've applied mascara, as the lashes may stick to the curler and come away with it! Always open the curler fully before taking it away from the lashes.

Mascara

Mascara, from an Italian word meaning 'to mask' or 'to hide', comes in many forms, but nowadays most of us tend to use a wand rather than the block form for ease of application. If this is your preferred choice of product then don't throw away old wands. Keep them clean and dry for separating your lashes in between coats. A word of warning here to contact-lens wearers: avoid mascaras with filaments, as they could fall off into your eyes and not only ruin your make-up and perhaps your lens, but cause considerable discomfort. If in any doubt then stick to allergy-tested mascaras or those sold by opticians as being especially kind to eyes.

To apply mascara, start with the bottom lashes. Bend your head forward and roll your eyes upwards to look in your mirror. Hold the brush vertically and, using even, downward strokes, work from the inside and coat the lashes several at a time. Allow them to dry, and if you need a second coat separate them first with an old, clean mascara wand before repeating the process. When it comes to your top lashes, lean your head well back and look down into your mirror. This time, hold the brush horizontally and use circular, upward-curving movements, curling the lashes as you coat them.

Mascara is available in some pretty startling colours these days as well as in the more traditional ones, but I would steer well clear of the blues and purples unless you are going for a young, strong, fashion-orientated look. Brown is usually the most attractive and the most natural colour to use, as grey can appear insignificant against eye colours, and black, though effective, can look too harsh against fair skin and hair.

Try strengthening and conditioning your lashes before putting on mascara by applying a thin film of castor oil or vaseline to them on a regular basis. When applying mascara, have a cotton bud and a little milk cleanser at the ready to remove any excess. If you think your mascara is too thick, touch it with the tips of your fingers to separate it while it is still damp.

False eyelashes

A word here about false eyelashes: like eyeliner they come and go with fashion trends, and for most of the time, I think they are unnecessary, but that it not to say that they aren't right for you. You can use very fine lashes to produce a natural appearance, emphasizing the thickness of the natural lash without it looking artificial, or use heavier ones for a more exaggerated look. Individual lashes can even be used to help correct eye faults and give lift to the eyes. If you are going to use them make sure they are clean, naturally curled and shaped to suit your eyes. Having already put on your eyeshadow and liner (this provides a base for the lashes), apply the false lashes firmly to the roots of the natural ones. You can either apply the adhesive straight on to the base strip of the lashes or put it on with an orange stick if the lashes are particularly light. Keep your eyes closed for a few seconds to allow the adhesive to set, then press the lashes firmly but gently into position with an orange stick and then check the inner and outer corners to make sure they are firmly attached. Losing one of your false eyelashes in a public place really is an unnecessary embarrassment! When the adhesive has set, attach the lower lashes and, if necessary, touch up any shadow or liner.

At this point I would like to repeat once again that the essentials of beauty come from within, and the most attractive eyes are the result of good health and the right amount of sleep. Smoky atmospheres and too much alcohol will make them so puffy and bloodshot that no amount of eye make-up will correct them.

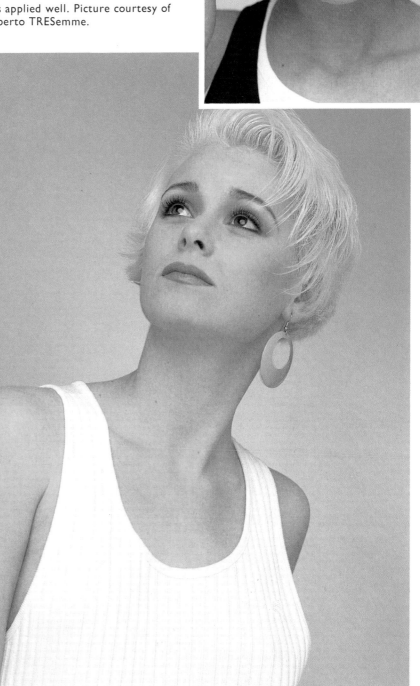

Essential for the application of mascara is a sure hand. Picture courtesy of Mary Quant. *Below:* There's no reason why blondes shouldn't wear dark mascara if it's applied well. Picture courtesy of Alberto TRESemme.

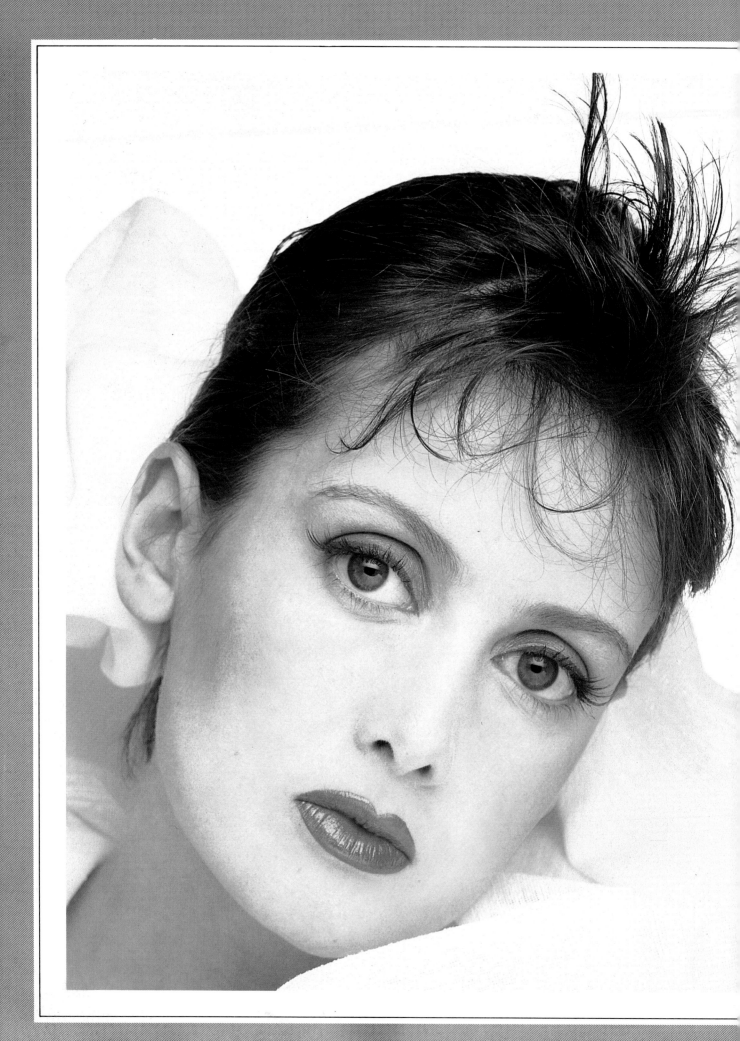

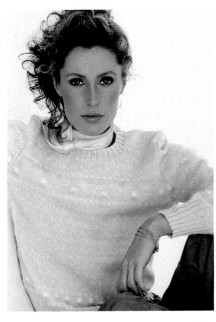 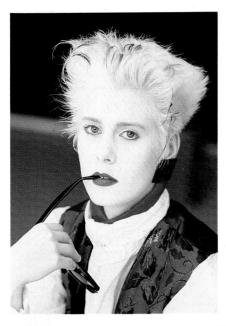

Main picture opposite: Pink shadow is complemented by bold blue eye liner to create this pastel effect from Christine at Mane Line.

Far left: Here a more traditional look has been achieved with mascara and eye liner. Picture courtesy of Mary Quant Cosmetics.

Left: Here Alan International have designed a face to match the hair. Pale lemony shadow combines well with the blonde hair, as does the contrasting brown liner and mascara with the darker spikes of hair. Matched to a light face, the end product is pale but certainly not insignificant!

Below: This picture from Stevie Buckle shows how face painting can be discreet. Here it has been done at the corner of the eyes.

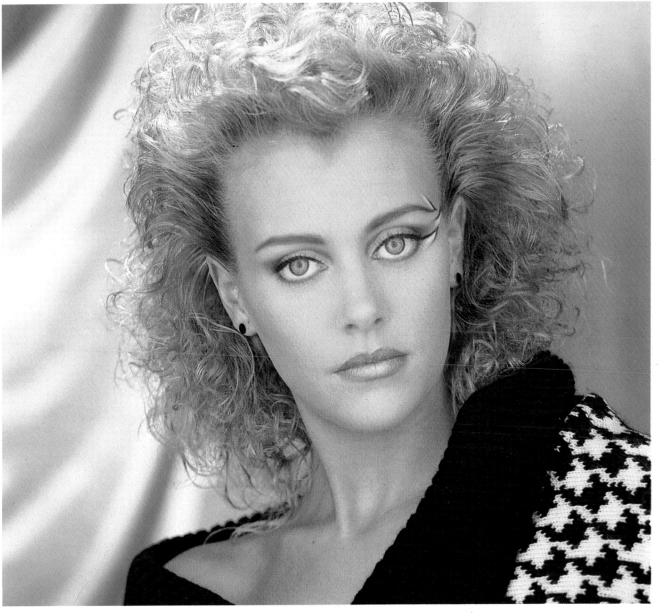

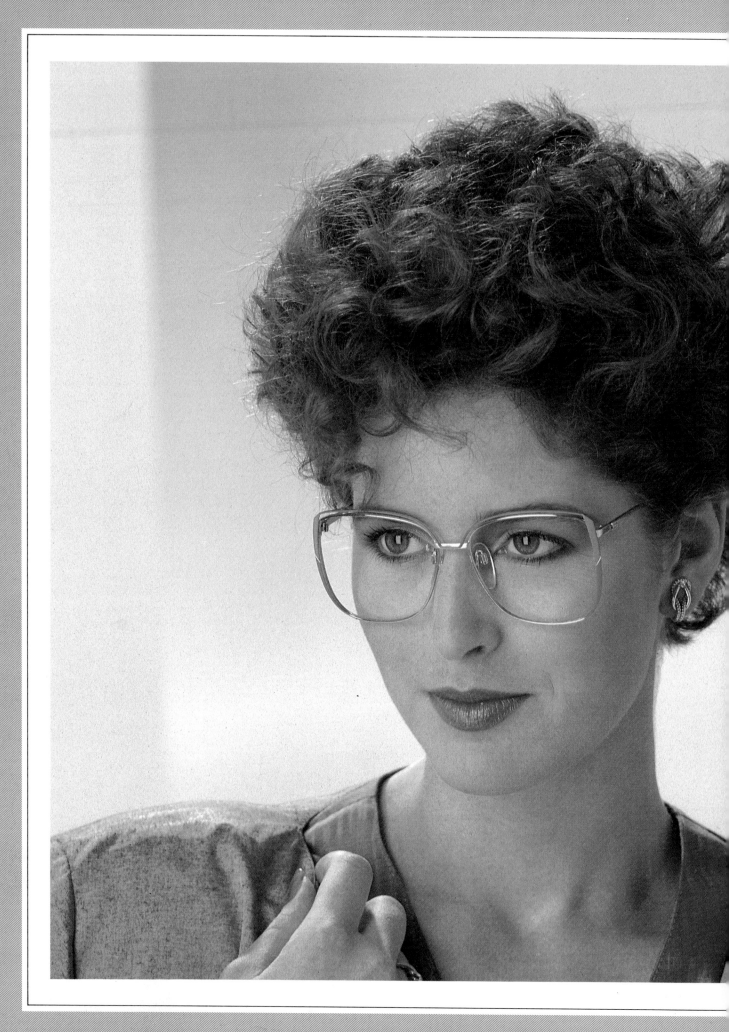

Positive thoughts for the short-sighted

Glasses

Crystal clear, beautiful eyes are something we all strive for, but many of us are handicapped by bad eyesight. It's easy to feel negative about your eyes if you have to wear glasses, but these days there really is no reason why, even if your sight is less than perfect, your eyes still can't be the focal point of your face. Spectacle wearers tend to feel at a disadvantage, believing that their glasses are ugly and their eyes aren't worth a second glance, but they couldn't be more wrong. Frame manufacturers have at last realized that glasses can be a fashion accessory as well as a physical necessity, and there are thousands of spectacle frames out there, in all shapes, colours and sizes, just waiting to enhance your wardrobe. With so much competition amongst manufacturers, prices have come down considerably, too, so now it's even possible to have two or three – or even more – pairs of specs, enabling you to ring the changes and provide accessories for a variety of different outfits!

There's no reason why girls who wear glasses shouldn't look as stunning as those who don't. Select your frames well and don't let them dominate the face. Above all, don't ignore your hair and make-up! Picture courtesy of Silhouette.

The main thing for spectacle wearers to remember about make-up is not to go from one extreme to another. You don't want to make your eyes look so overpowering that people don't see any other aspects of your face, which may be equally pleasing. Equally, you don't want your eyes to look insignificant under a too-magnificent pair of frames. There are a couple of golden rules here as far as specs wearers are concerned. The first one is to go for a first-class hairstyle which you know suits you. Limp, bedraggled hair, a heavy fringe with a nose and a pair of spectacles peeking out from under it isn't going to flatter anybody, but you'd be surprised how many people who wear glasses ignore their hair altogether.

The second rule is to always make up your face completely. Never ignore the lips or the blusher as, by doing so, you are going to create that very imbalance you should be trying so hard to avoid. Remember, too, that the effect of your make-up will vary according to the type of lenses you wear. Lenses for short-sightedness make the eye appear smaller, so you need to brighten the eyes and perhaps use more make-up than you normally would. Lenses for long sight, however, magnify the eyes, so don't go overboard – less is best.

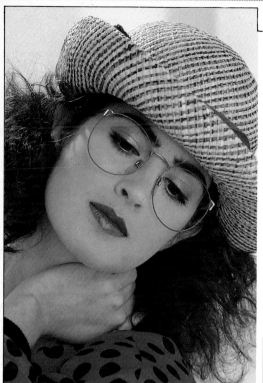

Contact lenses

Contact lenses have long since been a confidence boost for those of us with impaired vision and, whether your lenses are hard or soft, there is no reason why you shouldn't be applying eye make-up in much the same way as you would if your vision was perfect.

Why not sport different coloured frames to match your mood and your wardrobe? Spectacle frames are now reasonably priced so buy two or three and wear them as a fashion asset. Photographs courtesy of Silhouette.

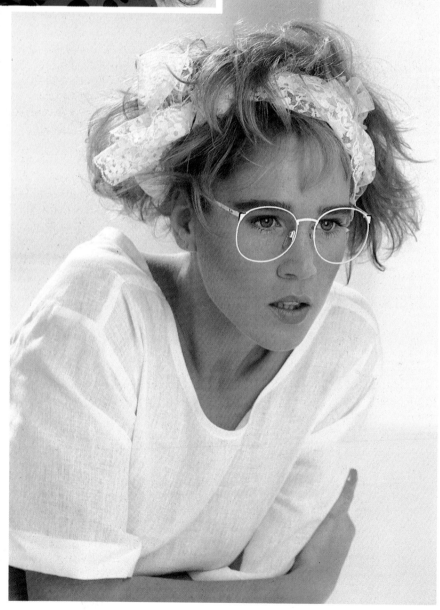

You do have to be extra careful, though, and keep everything scrupulously clean when applying make-up. At which stage you put your lenses in, before or after making-up, is really a matter of personal taste, and there are arguments for and against each method. Some manufacturers believe strongly that eye make-up should be applied after lens insertion to avoid contact with make-up, oil or other substances caught in the finger prints. This is a good point, but in the past I have found it easiest to put in my contact lenses last of all. In my experience they very easily attract powdery particles of make-up and, though you may not be immediately aware of their existence, this can have a build-up effect which will soil an otherwise perfectly good lens. Also, when you are applying make-up, particularly on the eye area, you tend to have your eyes wide open for a considerable length of time. As lenses need the moisture produced by the eye's continual blinking to keep them comfortable I have found that my lenses have felt dry, almost 'sticky' after I've finished applying my make-up, simply because of the length of time my eyes have been open. Your hands should always be scrupulously clean and thoroughly washed before you apply lenses anyway, so if there are any particles of product on your fingers they should end up down the sink and not in your eye!

As a veteran contact-lens wearer, I do feel that the best products to use around the eye area are allergy-tested and fragrance-free ones. Allergic reactions on the eyes always seem to affect those with poor vision much more drastically, and it's better to be safe than sorry. And always use a mascara without filaments, as these can break off the lashes and fall into the eyes. Any mascara which claims to be lash-lengthening probably has fibres in it, so avoid these at all costs.

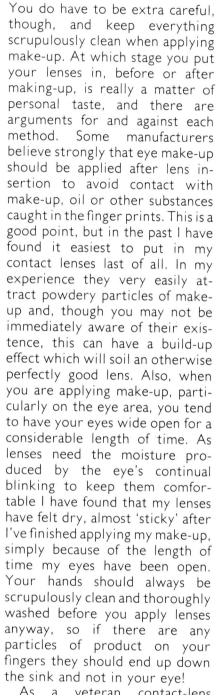

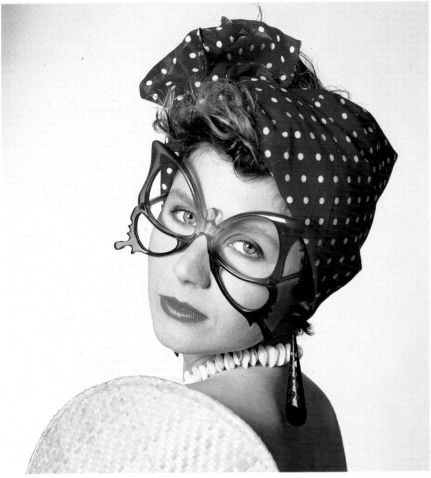

These frames from Pearle Vision show that specs can be fashionable and fun! Be careful with eye make-up if you wear flamboyant frames as you don't want to look overpowering, but neither do you want your eyes to pale into insignificance.

cation of mascara on the outer lashes. For eyes that are too far apart, begin the shadow close to the nose, as this will help focus on the inner corners. Shadow under the eye is a nice finishing touch and a good eye enlarger, but take it no further than the centre of the eye or the area will appear to decrease in size.

Make-up removal

When it comes to taking off your eye make-up you need to treat your eyes with an exceptional amount of tender, loving care. I would recommend buying a make-up remover by a known and well-established company which has gone to the trouble of producing a product especially for this delicate area. Avoid heavy creams or greasy lotions, as they will drag at your skin and make your eyes feel tired. Always take your lenses out before removing make-up. By not doing so you risk irritating your eye and tearing, scratching, and perhaps even losing your lens.

Look at your fingernails closely. If they are too long you are running a high risk of scratching or tearing your lenses, apart from the fact that they must be more difficult to insert. Try and avoid atomizers, but if they are necessary – hairspray for instance – use them before you put your lenses in. When it comes to applying eyeshadow, you want something that is going to stay fast. It should not be necessary to re-apply your shadow during the day, but this is even more relevant to contact-lens wearers, as you want to avoid fiddling with your eyes. Use powdered eye shadow with a dampened applicator, either a brush or a sponge, to ensure that the colour is well sealed on to the lids and to avoid powdery particles being flicked into the eye.

Eye make-up

The eye make-up hints and tricks mentioned in the previous chapters can be used by contact-lens and spectacle-wearers just as much as by anybody else. If you want to make your eyes look larger, and this particularly applies if you are short-sighted and wear glasses, recede the brow bone using a darker shadow and blend it well in an outward direction. Make your lashes look thicker either by dotting eye liner at the root of the lashes or by drawing a line and then smudging for a soft effect. If your eyes are too close together, then accent the outer corners. Start your shadow and liner at the centre of the lid and extend the shadow ever so slightly beyond the outer corners, with a generous appli-

Do's and Don'ts

Finally, here are a few general rules for all of us to avoid contamination of eye make-up. Never lend your eye cosmetics or borrow other people's, as that completely defeats the object of an allergic-tested product! To minimize contamination, buy tubes and self-applicators instead of open containers. The moment anything seems to irritate, then stop using it and consult your doctor. And never apply your make-up on the move. A sudden jolt, in a car for instance, might cause a sponge applicator or mascara brush to end up in the eye rather than being applied to the area around it, which is double trouble for contact-lens wearers.

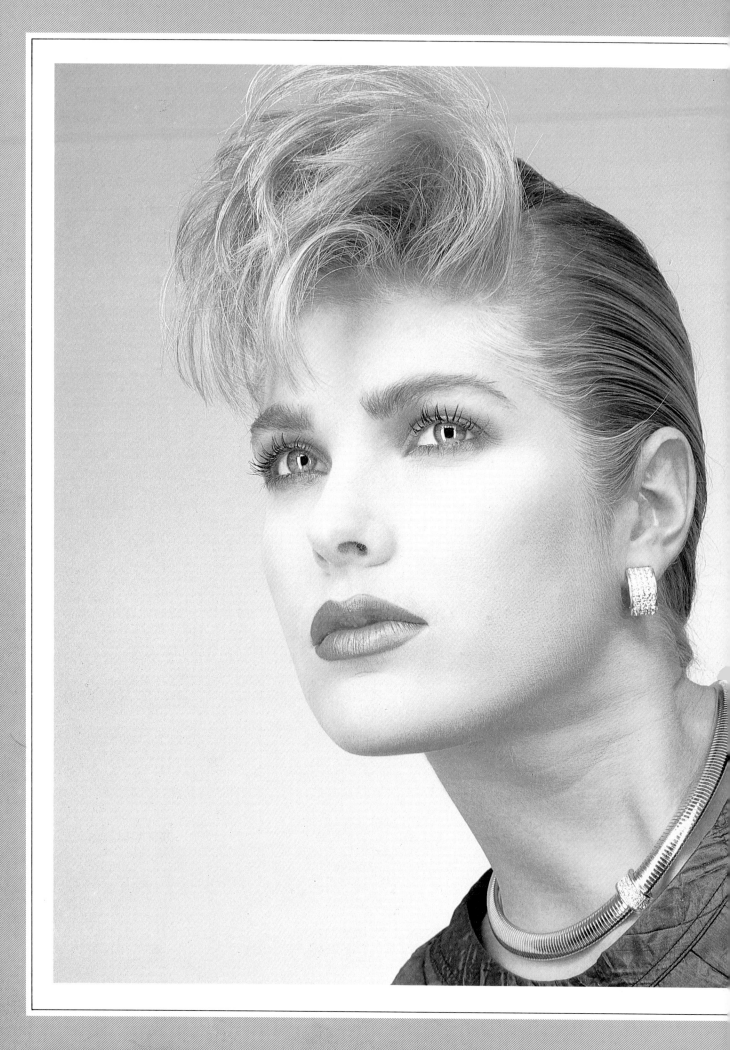

Sealed with a kiss

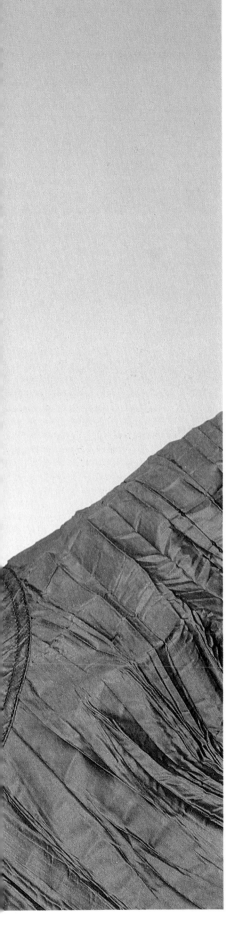

No matter how expertly you have applied the rest of your make-up, you will look unfinished, almost naked, without lipstick. The effect of lipstick is to pull the whole face together, to make it look complete, to harmonize your looks and give your face vitality. When not looking at your eyes, the people you meet during the course of a normal day are going to spend a great deal of time looking at your lips, so it would be a downright shame not to make the most of them.

Lipstick types

In its time, lipstick has appeared in many forms – gloss, creams, sticks, and crayons amongst them. There has been stay-fast, matt and oozing, glossy, and wet-look lipstick. It has even been white, black or completely transparent and tasting of strawberries! Many of these varieties have been fads, but lipstick does vary a great deal in texture and density, ranging from gloss, which is basically designed to top up your lip colour or to just add a hint of colour by itself, to the thicker, creamier variety which, once applied to your lips, is designed to stay there. The type you choose depends entirely on

No matter how hard you try to perfect the rest of your face, you'll look naked if you don't add the ultimate finishing touch – lipstick. Even here there are some golden rules to follow to make sure you look your best. Picture courtesy of Schwarzkopf.

you and your lifestyle. It may be that you don't mind frequently re-applying your lipstick or that, no matter how many tricks you use to help it stay on and how long-lasting it claims to be, it still needs frequent touching up.

Sadly, in the latter case, you are one of life's lip-lickers, and there's nothing, aside from changing your habits, that you can do about it. As a general rule, when you are testing lipstick, if it glides smoothly on to your hand and leaves only a slight stain when wiped off with tissue the colour will probably hold fast for some time. Lip gloss is made from a gel base and doesn't have any lubrication, so if your lips are dry they need the emollients contained in a lipstick – although, of course, you can put gloss on top. Lipsticks which are designed to stick around often make a good base, rather than the main shade, as the colour can otherwise be too heavy and dominant. Gloss over these with a gentler, more translucent tint. This way your lips will look slick and have colour sealed in.

Putting it on

If you apply lipstick without a brush, then you'll just look as if you've been smacked in the face – you can't possibly apply this make-up properly without the correct tool. The use of a brush, and even a lip-lining pencil, will give you a much clearer, defined line. It's also far more economical, as it forces you to handle your lipstick with care.

Start by dotting a little foundation on to the lips and smoothing it in; this will provide a good base on which to set the lipstick. Now take a pencil and draw a firm, clear line around the edges. This will help stop lipstick 'bleeding', or spreading into the skin around the lips. Use a pencil either in a natural tone for your skin and lip colour or one which complements your lipstick. I personally think a more natural tone is better if you know you are going to be in a situation where your lipstick will be coming off but you can't retouch it – a long business lunch, for instance. That way, when the colour fades you won't be left with a totally unnatural line around the outside of your mouth.

Now you can fill in your mouth with colour from your lipstick with a brush. Choose a fine one with a long handle for good leverage. You'll find that a cheap brush is likely to leave a trail of bristles on your lips, which will become embedded in the colour, and will be messy and time-consuming to take out. Collect the lipstick on to the brush in gentle sweeps, never taking too much, as you'll ruin the lipstick if you are heavy handed at this stage. Prop your elbow on the dressing table and look straight into the mirror. For even more stability, place your little finger on your chin, which will give you just enough movement in your thumb and forefinger to enable you to hold the brush properly but manoeuvre it well. Once you've applied the first coat of lipstick, blot with a tissue. Dab on a tiny amount of translucent powder to really seal in the colour and then apply another coat of lipstick. Blot again. Then top with your final coat or with gloss.

A word of warning: nothing looks more messy and unnatural than lipstick on teeth. Many women end up with more make-up inside their mouths than on

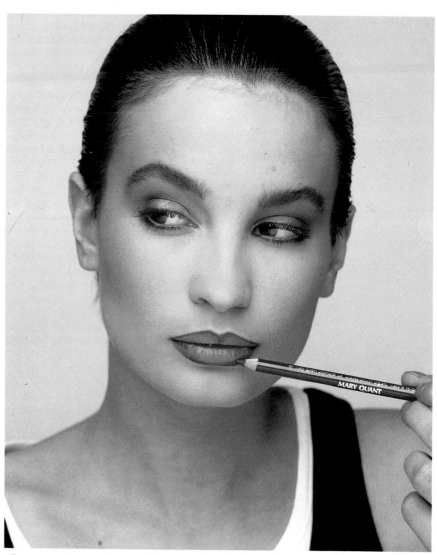

By using a lip pencil you will ensure that the lipstick colour won't bleed and that the shape of your lips will be well defined. Picture courtesy Mary Quant Cosmetics.

their lips – through no fault of their own. It might just be the way they laugh or the way in which their lips curl. Do check before you go out that this has not happened to you. Look in the mirror, smile, and talk to yourself. And don't be satisfied until your teeth stay white. If you think it is going to be a problem during the day, spread a little vaseline across your teeth with your fingertips. This will help the lips to glide over the teeth and not drag over them. Apply lipstick to just two-thirds of your lips, leaving the inner areas clear, and remember when you are applying your lipstick that the intensity of colour must balance with the rest of your make-up.

Apply lipstick last of all, after you have dressed, not only to avoid staining your clothes but also to get a better picture of your total image.

Enhancing and disguising

Like eyes, lips can be fully exploited or cleverly disguised with the aid of make-up. Wide lips can be made to look narrower if you first cover the edges of the mouth with foundation and draw an outline with your brush that ends before it reaches the corners. If you have thin lips that you want to make look bigger, carefully apply pale foundation around the outer shape of the lips. Outline the natural lip line with a pale-coloured lipstick, and fill in the shape with a slightly darker but toning colour. Soft colours are best here, as brighter ones make things stand out, and so will actually emphasize a thin lip shape. If you have what you consider to be a large mouth, use a subdued lip colour and pay special attention to the eyes and cheeks when making up so as to deflect attention from the lip area. To slim them down even more, outline your lips with a deep-coloured lip pencil just inside the lip line, as this will help you to keep the lipstick within the natural borders of the mouth.

Mismatched lips are quite a common problem, and can be easily remedied by using more than one lip colour. If one lip is bigger than the other use a slightly lighter shade on the smaller lip and a darker shade on the larger. Blend a little of the paler colour on to the centre of the fuller lip so that the difference is not discernible. It's important not to over-correct or you'll just be drawing attention to your fault. Try and remember that the days of cupid's bows really are over; it's much more flattering and far less dating to make the most of what nature has given you.

Lipstick has a protective, as well as a cosmetic, effect on our lips, which is just as well, because they certainly do need it but very easily get overlooked. All outside elements have a drying, chafing effect on lips and, just as you wouldn't dream of stepping into brilliant sunshine without protecting your eyes with sunglasses or your body with a barrier cream, so you should also protect your lips. If you are not wearing make-up at all, so that even a light smattering of gloss would look out of place, then wear a protective lip salve, barrier cream or even a little vaseline.

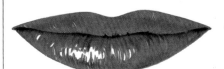

Ideal lips are well proportioned and a balanced size.

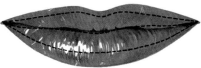

For thin upper lips, use a lighter shade of lipstick on the slim area to make it appear more full.

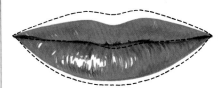

Apply foundation around the outer shape of thin lips, then add a pale coloured lipstick and fill in with a slightly darker colour.

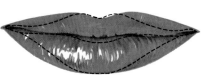

Here a lighter shade has been used on the thinner lower lip to make it appear a fuller shape.

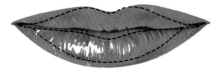

Reduce heavy lips by drawing the lip line just inside of their natural line and keeping the lipstick within these areas.

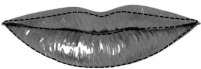

Lip liner can be discreetly used to give a better, more defined shape to lips which tend to be oval shaped.

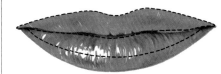

Cupid lips were once extremely popular but the days of the obvious cupid's bow are now well and truly over.

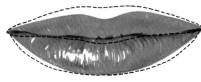

Lift a drooping lip with liner at the top edges of the mouth and fill them in with lipstick.

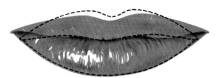

Take your lip liner just outside the boundaries of the lips if you consider them to be small and fill in with lipstick to these new limits.

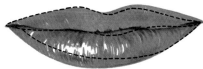

Lip pencil has almost magical qualities — it can even be used to correct uneven lips if applied with a steady hand.

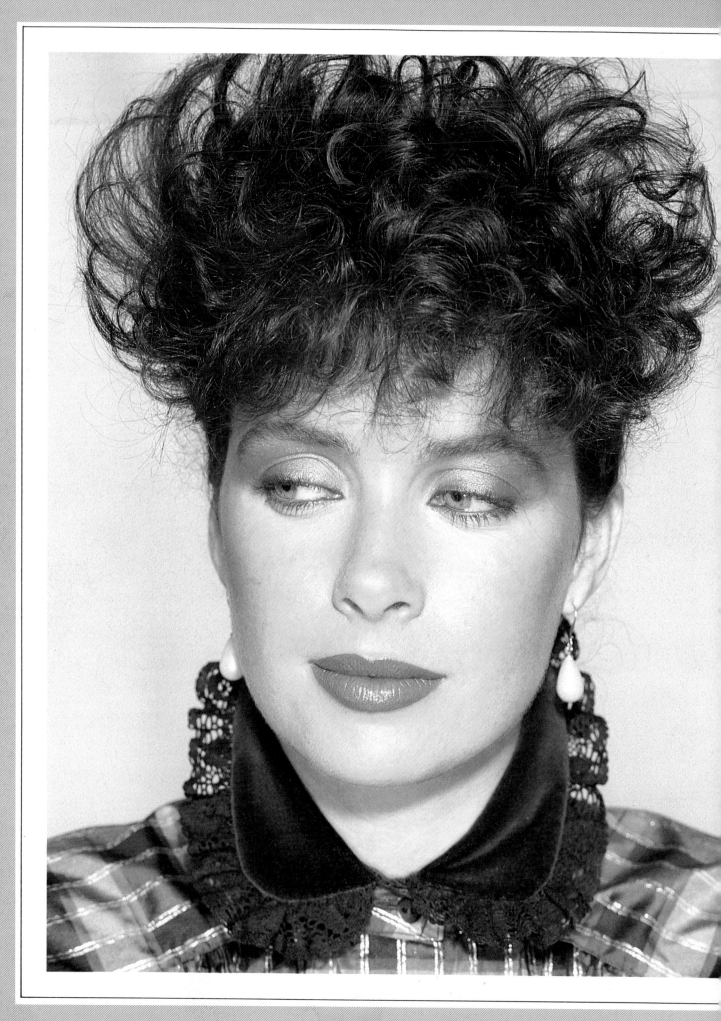

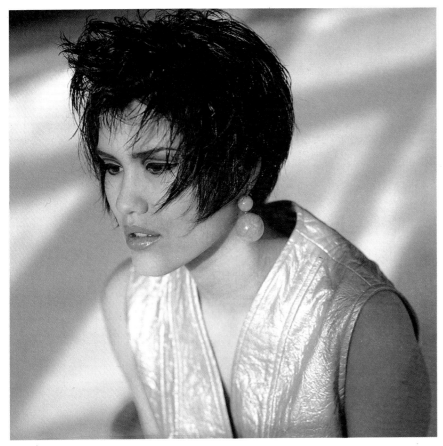

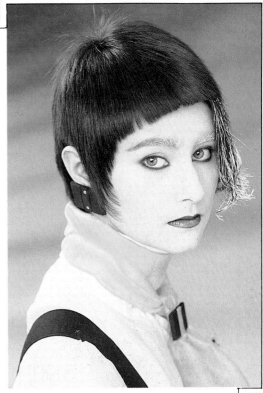

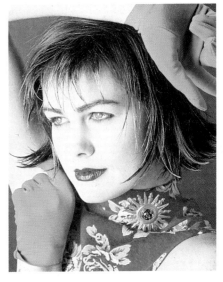

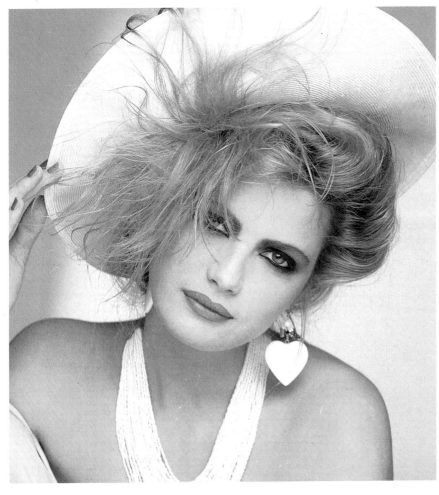

Pink lipstick has been discreetly topped with matching gloss to complete this pretty make-up statement which elegantly complements the mauve lines of the outfit. Picture courtesy of Schwarzkopf.

Top left: Even pale lipstick can be made to look interesting with the addition of lip gloss. Picture courtesy of Schwarzkopf.

Top right: Alan International have gone one step better by matching the lipstick to the eye liner and coloured streaks — is this the ultimate in mix and match make-up?

Bottom left: A creamy, matt pink/brown lipstick has been used by Christine at Mane Line for this soft, summery effect.

Above: True vibrancy is achieved with this bright red lipstick and matching dress from Boots No 17.

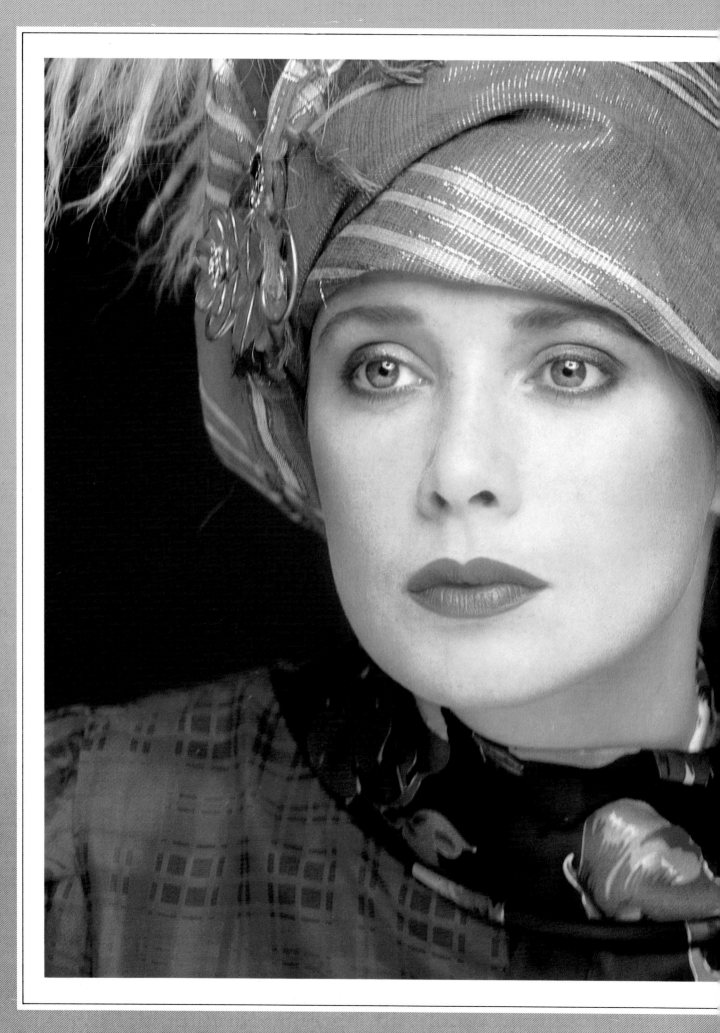

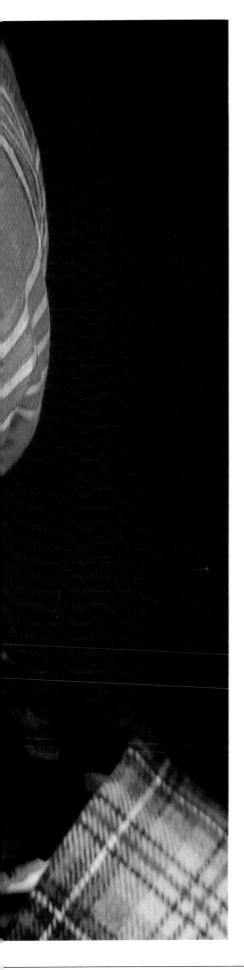

Stepping out and growing up in style

By now you should be mastering the art of make-up and should be adept at your morning routine. You should know how to apply it to make it last, and you should be able to put it on in less than 20 minutes. All very well, you may say, but what if there's a special occasion, surely that will take longer? Not necessarily. In the same way that a 'natural-looking' face does not necessarily take less time to create (you would still apply the same number of products, but perhaps less of them) you don't have to paint and preen for an hour in front of the mirror for a stunning night-time look.

Day into night

However, the chances are that, if you've had a hectic day and are going out straight from work or have to change first, your make-up will need touching up in some way to help you feel fresher and more alert. For the quickest day-into-night transformation, take a light tissue or a piece of cotton wool and gently buff off all your excess make-up to remove any of the dirt and grime your face is bound to have picked up during the day. Give your face a fresh application of powder all over, apply a little more blusher, re-apply lipstick and hey presto!

Remember that, although you can get away with bolder colours at night – electric light is less harsh than daylight – you don't necessarily want more of them. Layers of make-up under strong artificial lights can actually look quite unpleasant. Go for less texture but bolder colours; it's brightness you want rather than quantity. Use pinkier, rosier colours in the softer lights of a candelit restaurant, as beiges turn grey in this kind of light. Your face needs to be illuminated at night, otherwise it will look flat, but don't go over the top with shininess. Illuminate only where the skin seems to want it, with perhaps a little highlighter on the brow bone for shimmer rather than shine. Analyze your daytime make-up and see where it can be enlivened. If, for instance, you normally wear a grey eye shadow and a palish lipstick, try blending in a little sapphire, not necessarily all over the lid but perhaps just on the outer corners, and use a bolder, deeper lip colour. The golden rule for night is: less is more. Take a long lingering look at your eye make-up before you re-apply. If you aren't adding any

Believe it or not, with a little bit of time in the ladies after work, you can transform your daytime look into something as stunning as this straight from work! Christine at Mane Line has used a head wrap for extra glamour.

extra hints of colour, do they really need touching up? If the make-up has creased or faded away very badly, then you are either using the wrong product for you or perhaps you are not applying it properly.

The natural look

At the other end of the scale is that natural, no make-up look that at some time or other most of us want to achieve, perhaps because we lead sporty lives or are going to spend the day in the country. For whatever reason, the naturally made-up look should never be seen as a soft option. Only in the summer, when you exude a glow of health and vitality, and your skin may be darker and your hair lighter, can you really get away with just a smattering of mascara and a touch of lip gloss. For those of us who refuse to bare our faces to the sun but still want to get 'back to nature', the skilful art of a 'naturally' made-up face is an essential one to master. When you put on your 'natural' face you are probably going to be using just as many products as you would for, say, a work day, but you are going to be more deliberate about their application. You still have to keep a good balance of colour, but what your are aiming for is a less intense result. If you have an imbalanced face your make-up will not look natural, just unfinished, so wear a paler blusher, maybe a rose pink instead of a red pink, or apply less than normal. And stick to paler lipsticks or just lip gloss and neutral, earthy-toned eye shadow colours. Out goes the azure and cobalt blue, in come the bronzes, creams and apricots.

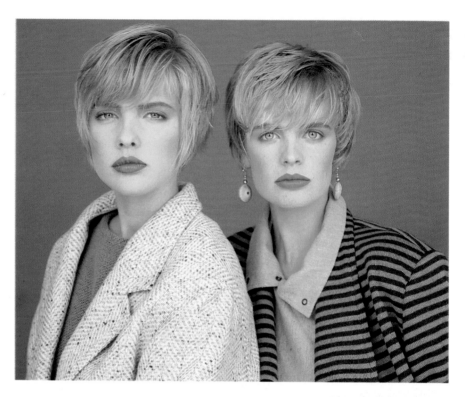

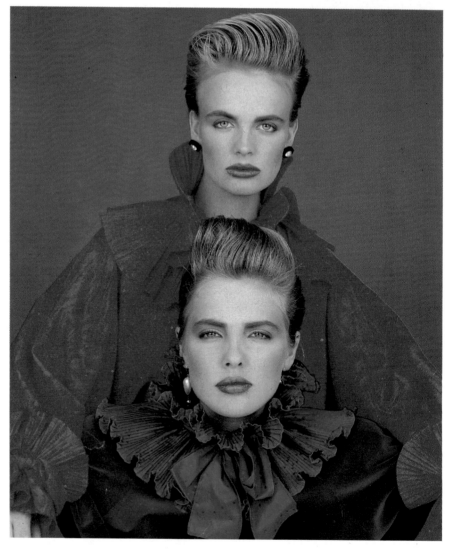

Two fine examples of how a day make-up can be wonderfully transformed for a night on the town. Almay has created these looks with the help of styling aids for the sleek hairstyles and their Mixed Doubles product range.

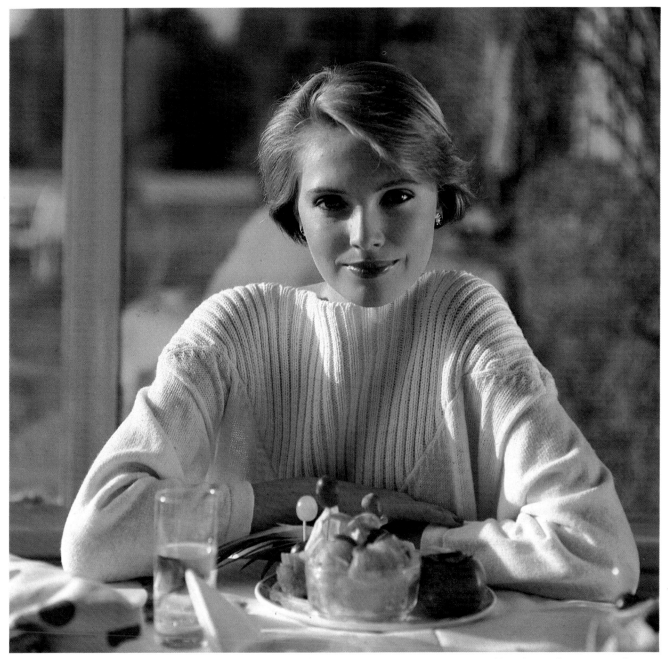

Make-up can be as discreet as it can be positive. You probably wouldn't want to look too well made-up, for instance, for a day out in the country. A well-balanced diet is also important for a naturally radiant face. Picture courtesy of Almay.

Once in a lifetime

The one occasion when a woman really can be forgiven, if not actively encouraged, for paying special attention to her face and make-up is her wedding day. Those wedding-day photographs are going to live with you forever, so it's up to you to do everything within your power to ensure you look your best – and maybe from those efforts you'll pick up habits which will last a lifetime. Start preparing your skin at least a couple of weeks before the big day, preferably a month. Make exfoliation (see page 29) part of your regular, daily skin-care régime, as this will help liven up what might have become a dull complexion. If you intend to invest in a facial (and professionally done ones are very relaxing), then do so at least five days before the wedding, as the facial and stimulating face-pack will bring out any little spots which might have been lurking under the surface of the skin.

Now for the make-up. If ever there was a time to invest in a once-over from a professional make-up artist then it's now. It's worth every penny to make sure that you look your very best for this special day, and you may discover things about your face that you've never previously realized! Make sure it is a make-up artist you visit, though, rather than a beautician in a beauty salon.

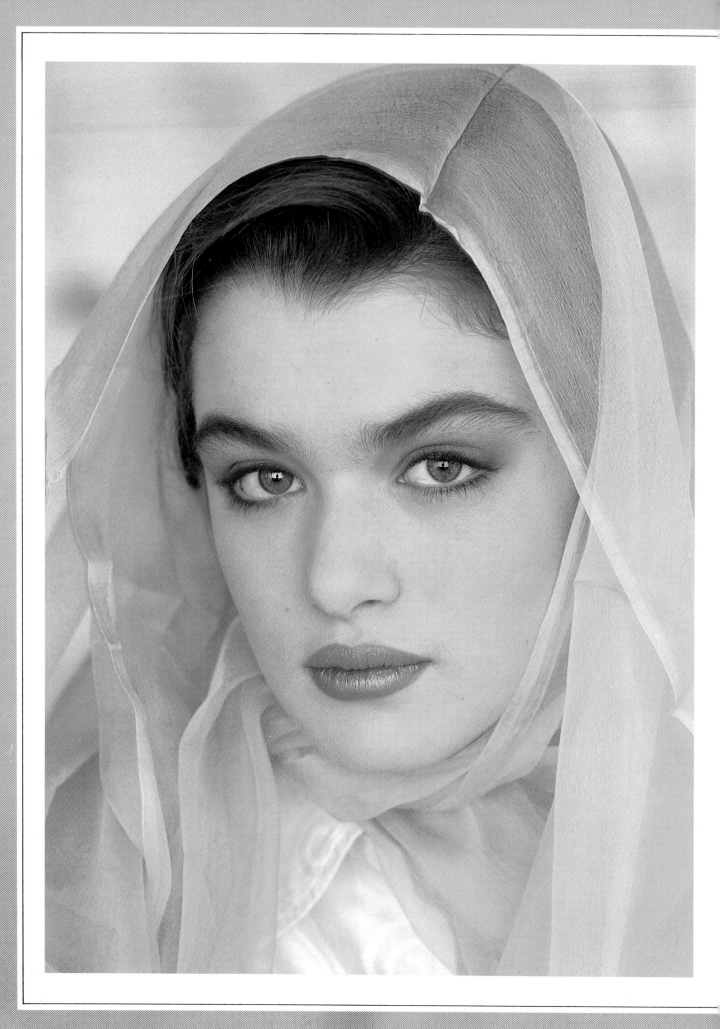

Beauticians are trained in the art of make-up application, and are certainly adept at it, but it is not what they are doing for a living all day and every day. Go to someone who specializes and who knows their craft thoroughly. Visit them, or start creating your face for yourself, about a week or two before the wedding and then repeat the look several times, so you know you've got it off to a fine art. Keep the look simple, clean and light, with no strong colours. Browns don't photograph well, and a bride should be creating the illusion of spring freshness, so light purples, lilacs, pale blues and apricots are best. As you are going to be photographed frequently, a matt look is preferable (the camera will exaggerate any highlights), so keep your loose translucent powder in a handy place in order to prevent any shine, and perk up your make-up as the day wears on.

Time and change

Up until this stage in your life the sky has virtually been the limit as far as make-up colours and techniques are concerned. Virtually anything goes as long as it suits you. It does pay, every six months or so, to reassess your make-up, to throw out what you don't use and to take a look at what is new to see what might suit. As you grow older this constant reassessment will pay dividends because, as your face ages, however slightly, it needs a change of make-up. At around the mid-30s, for instance, eyes start to need definition rather than an abundance of colour. Soft, smudgy, neutral colours like deep purples and browns are good, and hold within their colour ranges a host of different tones. The most common mistake

A bride's make-up needs to be soft and radiate a look of spring freshness and pretty pastel colours. This look was created by Molton Brown using their Sea Pearl range of cosmetic colours.

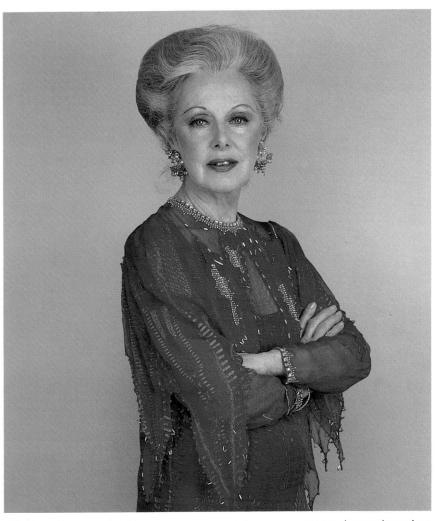

The last thing you should do as you mature is to stop wearing make-up altogether, it just needs to be adapted to your changing skin and to be applied more lightly and gently than before. Picture courtesy of Max Factor.

most women make as they get older is simply to stop wearing make-up altogether just because they don't know what to do. This is a mistake, as your face will lose all the definition it needs. What you should do is apply your make-up more lightly and gently than before. As skin ages it grows disorganized in pigment and texture, and foundation and powder help to pull it all together. Loose powder is an essential re-texture. Use it generously, and fluff off any excess with a brush or damp tissue. Blushers and highlighters should be placed only where the skin is smooth and tight. Avoid using any make-up with a yellow cast and keep it light and sheer, rather than bright. Eyes tend to narrow as they get older, so use a

shadow tone or sheer shade rather than a distinct colour. Upward strokes make the eyes look younger than lines that droop, so wash colour over the whole eyelid, blending it outwards and upwards towards the temples. And avoid browns, since they tend to bring down the eye.

For the softest lid shade, pencil a circle of colour in the palm of the hand, then apply it with your fingers on to the lid. The creaminess works as a soothing base for other eye make-up. And nothing reveals a woman trapped in time more than her eyebrows. Elderly-looking eyebrows tend to be either pencil-thin or super-straggly, while young eyebrows are soft, neat, well groomed and face-framing.

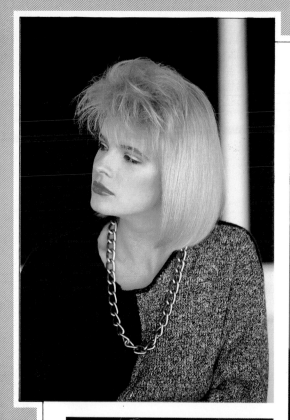

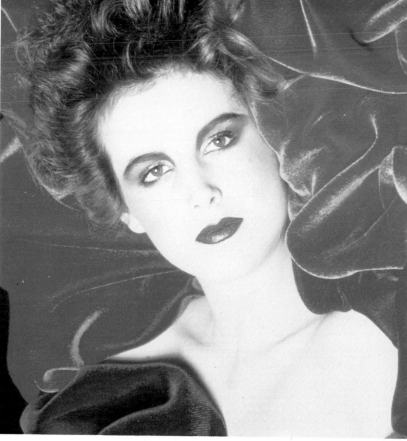

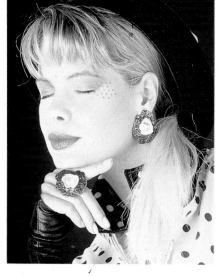

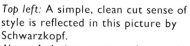

Top left: A simple, clean cut sense of style is reflected in this picture by Schwarzkopf.

Above: A daring, young and vampish Madonna look from Boots No 17.

Top right: An ultra glamorous yet classical Dior look.

Right: Strong colour statements are often needed to make short, casual hairstyles look more positive. Picture courtesy of Molton Brown.

Opposite: Strong definite colours make this make-up a sure fire hit for parties. Picture courtesy of Alan International and Quote Salons.

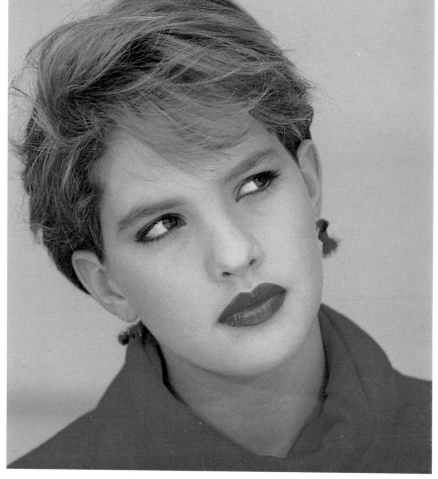

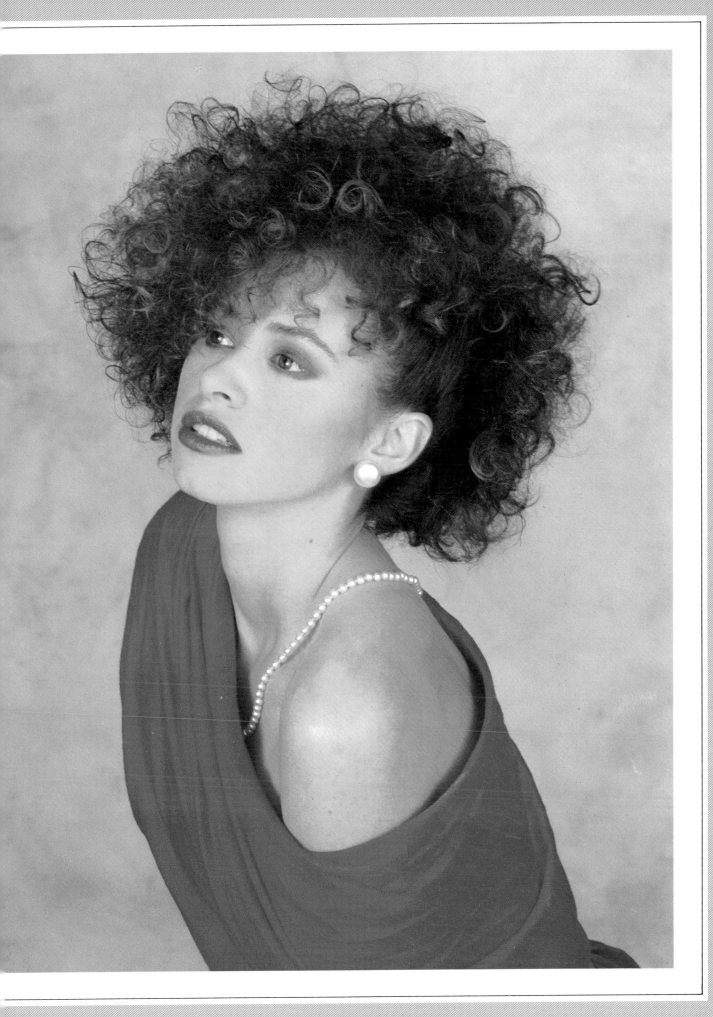

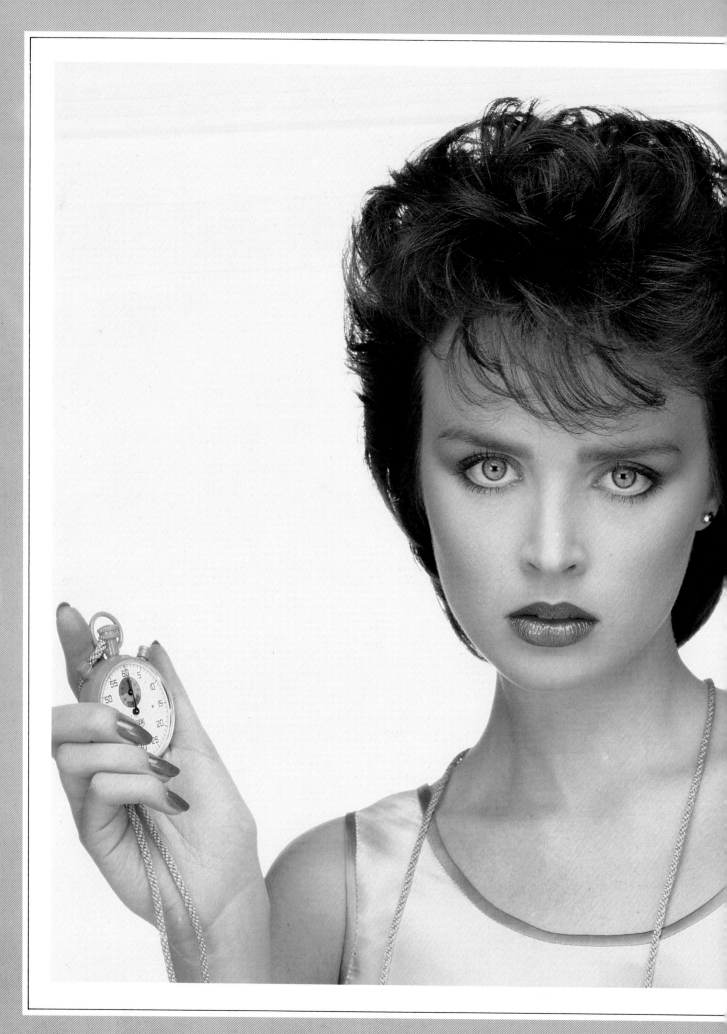

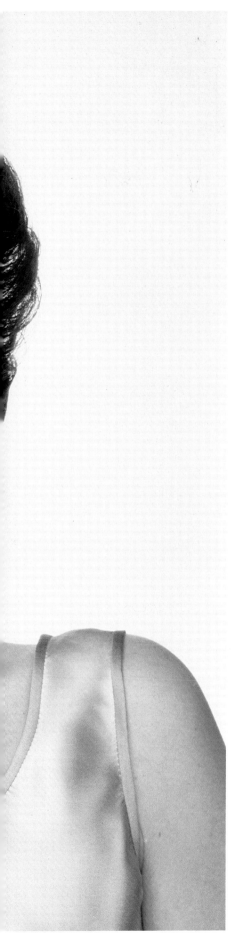

Hints, tips and 'wrinkles'

For easy reference, here is a list of do's and don'ts and time-saving hints to help you look your very best if you are in a hurry.

1 Before you consider applying any make-up to your face, get to know your skin type and tone and make sure you choose the correct base. Try at least two shades of base; it's the nearly invisible one you ought to go for.

2 Elimate shadows and tiny lines before you apply your make-up base by using a thin film of concealer on the affected areas. Apply it with a thin lip brush for extra accuracy.

3 When applying foundation, moisten your fingers with water as you move towards the chin line so that it blends out invisibly and leaves no lines. Nothing looks worse than seeing a rim of foundation around the jaw line. Try the same trick at the hairline, too.

4 Make-up applied too thickly only emphasizes lines. Tip it on to the centre three fingers and apply it in sweeping strokes over large areas and blend, blend, blend.

5 A harsh blob of blusher on the centre of the cheeks looks terrible, but for some people, knowing exactly where to apply it is a

You may think that to achieve a flawless make-up finish like this is an impossible task with so many rules to abide by. But once you have learnt the basic skills the key is flexibility. Picture courtesy of Mary Quant Cosmetics.

problem. Never bring cheek blusher closer to your nose than the outer rim of the iris of your eye or below the base of the nostrils. Draw an invisible line from the nostril base to the edges of your face and downwards from the rim of the iris. Apply blusher within this area – even on earlobes for extra evening allure.

6 A 'double blush' technique will ensure that blusher has real staying power. Apply a gel or sheer liquid blusher first, and then build on it with cream or powder blusher, depending on skin type.

7 When applying powder blusher, load your brush with it and then blow it off so that only the merest colour remains. This will ensure a light look.

8 Blend blusher high, from the upper cheekbones to the temples and hairline, to lift the face.

9 As a boost for a tired face, brush on colour lightly along the top of the forehead, under the chin and over the bridge of the nose. If your eyes look weary, wing the colour out to the temples and in again just above the eyebrows.

10 To avoid an over-made-up look, use a loose powder one shade darker than your normal one for contouring. A fluff of dark powder, for instance, makes a wonderful camouflage for the under-the-chin area.

11 Lid washing conceals flaws, unifies colour and texture and prepares the skin to accept and

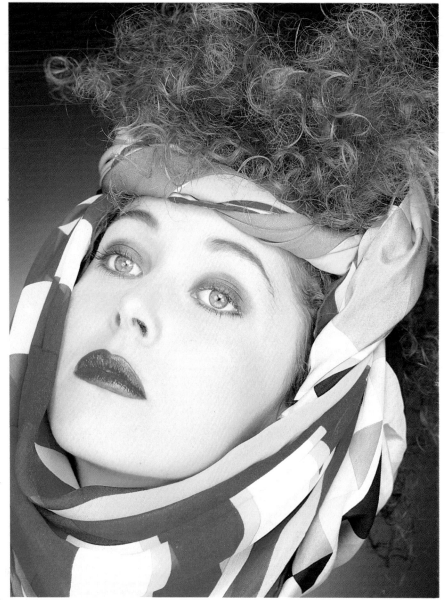

This beautifully bold look speaks volumes of fun without being too outrageous. The use of pencils around the eyes and expertly applied lipstick have worked extremely well here. Picture from Christine at Mane Line.

15 When you stroke on mascara, be sure to coat the eyelashes all the way to the tips. For a lavish look, coat the tips first, then brush up from underneath to curve the lashes slightly. Or, better still, use an eyelash curler before you apply mascara.

16 Always wait between applying coats of mascara. If a second coat is applied on top of a tacky one the lashes will become stuck together and look stiff and spiky.

17 For long-lasting lip colour, fill in the entire surface with a base coat of lip pencil. The matt cover prevents colour bleeding, and gives lipstick longer wear and a more interesting depth of texture.

18 To avoid getting loosened eye make-up in eyes, wrap your fingers in a tissue, moisten lashes with remover and, keeping the eye closed, gently sweep underside of lashes with the tissue, then down over the lids and lastly the lash tops.

19 For economy and flexibility, make one product do the work of two or three. A brown eye pencil, for instance, ·might not just be handy for tidying up the shape of the eyebrows; if soft enough it could also be used to outline eyes and lips. If you are really in a jam a toning brown eye shadow could be blended over the eyelids and then used sparingly as a face shader.

20 Never touch up your make-up in public. It not only looks sloppy and unhygenic, but also makes you appear to be obsessed with your looks. You want to carry your make-up with ease and confidence, so always retreat to the ladies' room to powder your nose.

hold colour. So include your eyelids in your make-up base.

12 Creamy, precise eye pencils are miracle workers. Try filling in the lower outside corner of your eye with a pencil and blend the line inward. Then hold your lid with your finger and pencil in deeper colour near the top lashes. It makes a good start for eye make-up and has the subtlest of effects. For a soft, translucent shadow colour, make a circle of pencil in the palm of your hand and, with one clean finger, work the pencil cream on to the whole lid.

13 When in doubt, smudge. A soft blur of colour takes less work, enhances any eye shape and looks softer.

14 Apply powder eye shadow wet and dry for longer-lasting and different effects. Powder eye shadow can be used as an eyeliner if applied wet, as it will go on two or three shades darker than it appears in the palette. Apply the same shadow, with a clean brush, dry, over the eyelid, and you will have achieved a subtle yet very pleasing blend of harmonizing colours.

Most women have a certain something which makes them feel totally dressed. It might be a pair of gloves, earrings or a hat. In this case, it's perfume and it is nice to finish your total look by smelling as good as you appear. Picture courtesy of Max Factor.

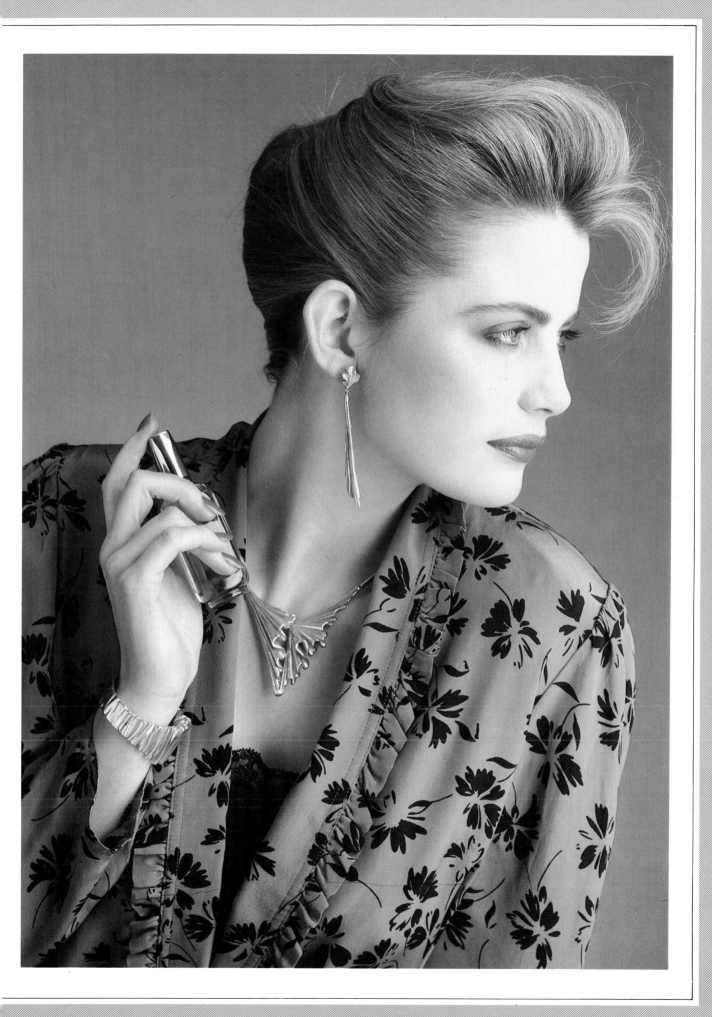

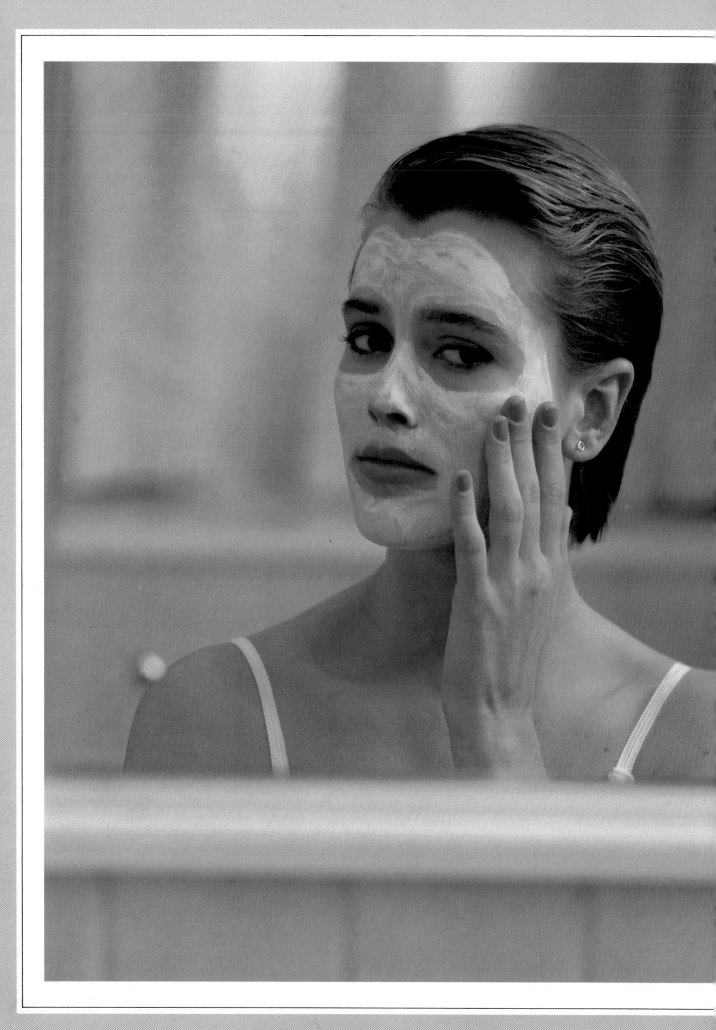

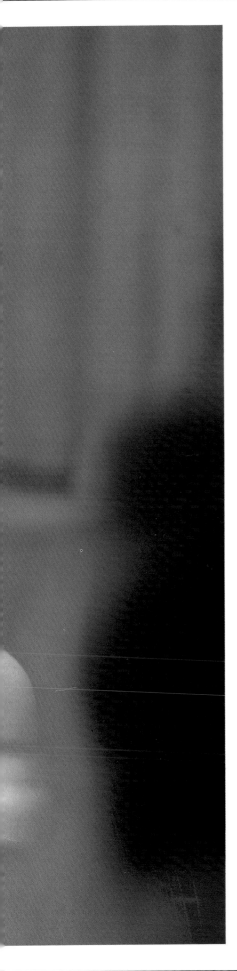

Make-up removal and skin treats

Long before reaching this page you should have discovered skin-care products and a routine which is right for you. We have already discussed the various cleansers and how they perform, so let's now go into a little more detail about how they should be put to work.

Cleansing

When it comes to taking off make-up at the end of the day, it never ceases to amaze me how slapdash people can be. Once or twice a year I am tempted to retire for the night without taking off my make-up, but I always wake up the next morning feeling stale, dirty and sloppy. There's also something about make-up on the pillowcase that I find repugnant: Proper cleansing is not only essential for the maintenance of good skin, but it is part of a routine and a self-discipline which is reflected in the way you look and the opinions other people form of you. So next time you've had a gruelling day and find yourself slipping into that 'couldn't be bothered' state of

A face mask won't magically improve your skin overnight but it is a good pick-me-up. Read this chapter first though, and make sure you choose a mask suitable for your skin type. Picture courtesy of Almay.

mind pull yourself together and consider. If a make-up-free skin which has done nothing more than spend a day in the fresh, clean air of the countryside needs to be efficiently cleansed, how dirty must a face be with at least two layers of beauty preparation and city grime on it?

Always remove any eye and lip make-up first to avoid spreading the cosmetics on these areas to other parts of the face. Be particularly gentle with your eyes, as the skin around them is very finely textured and the eye can be easily damaged. Use a clean tissue for each eye, so that if there is any trace of an infection in one it doesn't spread to the other, and use soft, gentle actions rather than ones which drag the skin. The worst thing you can do is clean off your eye make-up with soap and water or baby oil, which is heavy and will sting the eyes. You should use a product which is designed specifically for the eye area. Place a small amount of the remover on your tissue and lift it over the eyelashes and eyebrows very gently, then sweep it downwards and outwards repeatedly until all the eye make-up is removed. To make sure that you remove all traces of lipstick, pass a damp tissue gently across the lips from one corner to the other and then repeat the process from the other side using a clean tissue.

The way you clean your face, of course, depends on the method of cleansing and the product you have chosen. But do make sure that your hair is well off your face, preferably held back with a large band, as you don't want to get your hair covered in the cleansing agent, and you can't possibly cleanse properly if you have to continuously hold back hair with one hand. Watch out, too, for harsh tissues or cotton wool which could scratch the face. Your face is only clean when there is absolutely no evidence of make-up on your cotton wool so, if there is still just a trace left, repeat the cleansing routine all over again.

Skin treats

For those of us who have the time I think it's nice, just once a week, to pamper ourselves with a mild home-beauty treatment. Take extra long in the bath, manicure and paint your fingernails, and take special care when removing your make-up, perhaps even gently massaging the face with upward, circular strokes.

Face masks

What better way to top off an evening of total self-indulgence than a face mask? The contribution face masks actually make to beautiful skin is debatable since, like anything else, they cannot penetrate the skin beneath that dead surface layer, but they do stimulate and refresh the skin and are an ideal bedtime treat for tired or overworked faces.

There are three types of face mask, and it's as important to know which one is right for you as it is to recognize your skin type. There is such an exotic array of facial treats in shops these days that it's far too easy to buy one because it looks and sounds nice, only to find that it either does nothing for you or, worse still, causes a violent reaction. There

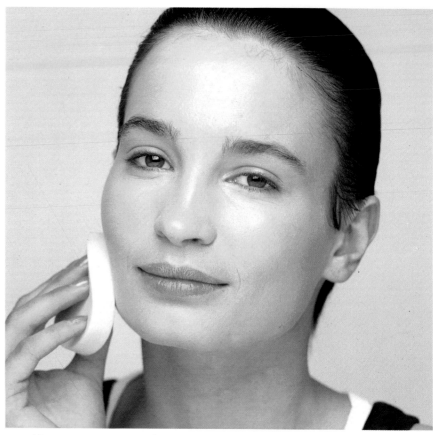

Always remove your make-up before going to bed. Make sure your skin is absolutely clean by looking at your cotton wool pad before you throw it away. Not until it's completely clear is your skin free of dirt. Picture courtesy of Max Factor.

are three main categories: setting masks, which include clay, sulphur, peeling and astringent masks; non-setting masks, which include those which are fruit, plant, herbal or vegetable-extract-based and those which contain 'natural' products, like fruits and honey and oatmeal, and, finally specialized masks, which include thermal, hot-oil and paraffin-wax masks.

Clay masks, which come within the first category, have basic ingredients like calamine, kaolin and fuller's earth. Calamine is the mildest of these, kaolin brings about a stronger response and fuller's earth an even more powerful one. Their active ingredients include rosewater, which has a mild toning effect, orange-flower water, which is stimulating, witch hazel, which is both stimulating and drying, and almond oil, which is used in a mask when a stimulating but not very

drying effect is desired.

The sulphur, peeling and stringent masks, also in the first category, are far more active than clay masks. While they set and tighten, the dead horny layer of the skin and oily secretions combine with the mask so that when the mask is removed, the old skin and the oil are removed as well. This has an especially drying effect on the skin, theoretically helping the control of blocked pores and blackheads. Setting masks are particularly good for younger skin types which will benefit most from their cleansing, toning and stimulating effect.

Although non-setting masks, the second category, form a film over the face which becomes firm and dry they do not have a tightening effect on the skin, nor do they affect its moisture content. This also means that your face doesn't become immobile while the mask is on. All masks

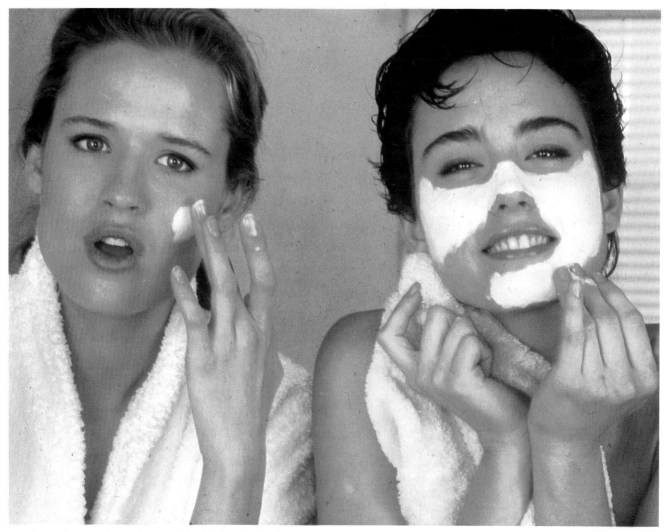

Some face masks set hard and feel tight while others are much lighter on the face. As with cleansing and moisturizing products, only certain masks will suit your skin, so choose your product carefully. Picture courtesy of Vichy.

which contain ingredients from natural sources rather than chemical ones are classed as biological, and they are ideal for sensitive skin, dehydrated or dry skin and skin congestion. Fruit masks are of this type. They have a stabilizing action on the skin's pH (see page 44), and water level. A combination of plants and fruit is ideal when the complexion is sluggish and needs to be stimulated as well as deeply cleansed. Herbal and vegetable masks offer the greatest choice of action. Cucumber works well on sensitive, delicate skin, while rosemary is a good tonic for a dry, dehydrated complexion. Herbal and seaweed products offer a gentle way of treating a blemished complexion without flaking or irritating the skin.

Specialized masks, the third category, are mainly confined to the beauty salon, since such things as hot-oil and paraffin masks are treatments for specific problems and need electrical apparatus for their application. There are warm masks, though, which have been modified in recent years and have become available as peel-off masks to use at home. These are designed to regenerate the skin, are said to delay the formation of surface lines, and are ideal for dry or mature skins.

Tonics

Toning should help complete your beauty routine both morning and night, and particularly after a face mask. There are skin tonics which gently tone the skin and remove

all traces of oil, grime and make-up. These are suitable for delicate, dry or mature skins. Astringents have a more stimulating, drying action and are for oily, coarse skins which are not sensitive, since astringent removes surface oil which can, in turn, disturb the skin's pH balance. Corrective lotions dry and heal the skin and remove oily matter from its surface. These are usually chemical formulations for badly blemished skins. After toning, the skin should feel slightly tacky to the touch and be calm and stable in appearance. Once the toner is completely dry, you are ready for a good night's rest or, at the start of the day, to apply some fresh make-up and start the cycle all over again!

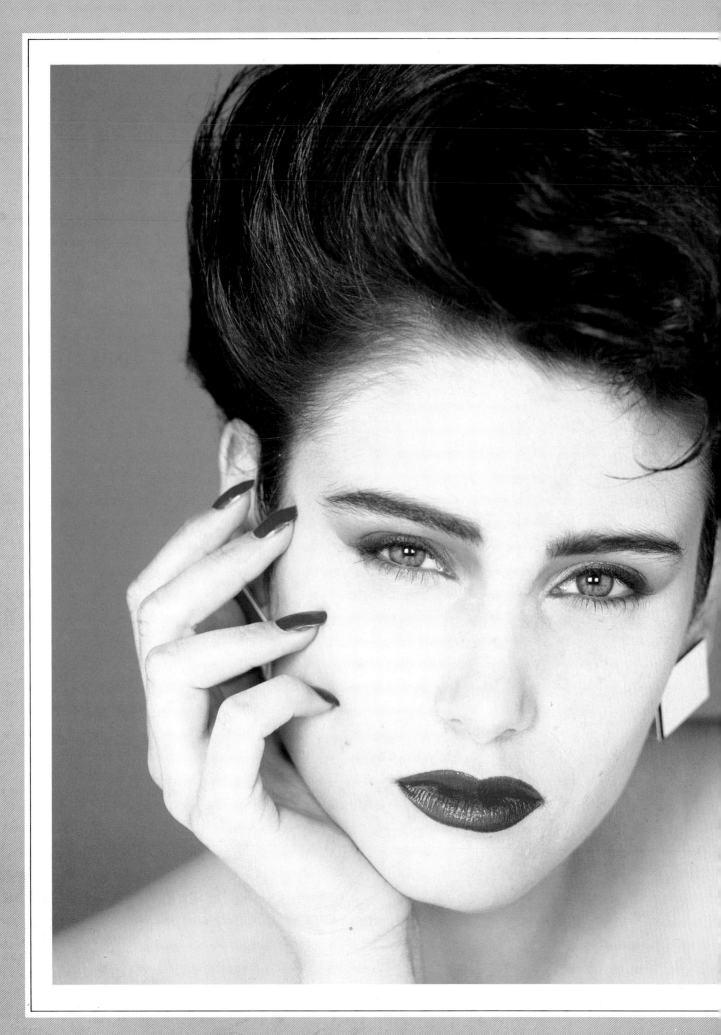

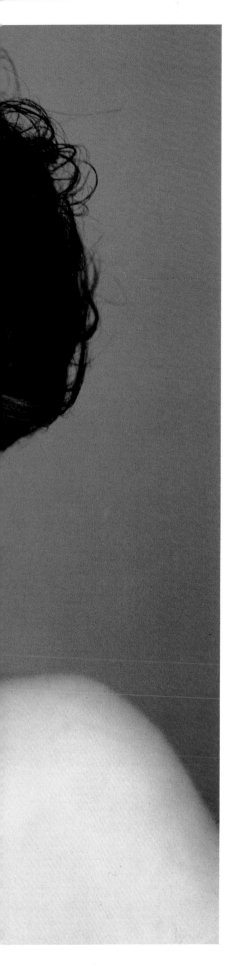

Good looks on the nail

I am sure you must have noticed that some women can spend a fortune on their clothes, yet still look as though they have been dragged through a hedge, while others can spend quite small sums of money on their attire and look a million dollars. Obviously if a woman is gifted with natural good looks she has a head start, and a sense of style helps too. But more than anything else what shows in a well-groomed woman is that she cares about herself. And caring about the way she looks means paying attention to small details, from the top of her head to the tip of her toes. One of life's real give-aways, and one that distinguishes sloppiness from sophistication, is fingernails. The most beautifully made-up, well-dressed woman in the world can be sadly let down by dirty, jagged and perhaps bitten fingernails. Think of how many things you do with your hands, how constantly they are on show. You eat with them, drink with them, work with them and animate your conversation with them. So, having worked to present a first-class image of ourselves to the public, it would be absurd to let that image down. Nicely manicured nails can also do a great deal to enhance that total look and complete the picture, as nail colour can be matched up to lipstick, make-up and clothes.

Structure of the nail

The nail's main role is as a protector, safeguarding the sensitive areas of our fingers and toes. The fact that it can be dressed up to suit our lifestyle is a bonus for us. It is an appendage of the skin, and includes a nail plate and the tissue that surrounds it. The part of the nail which is visible is the nail plate, which is the hard keratin portion on the top of the finger. The nail bed is the area of tissue directly underneath the nail plate.

If a nail looks pink then it is healthy, as this means the blood is flowing to the nail bed and can be seen through the nail plate. The free edge of the nail is the part beyond the edge of the fingertip which is visible from both sides of the hand. The surrounding part of the nail is made up of the following tissue. The cuticle is a thin semi-circular piece of skin that overlaps the nail. The eponychium is the inside point where the nail enters the skin. The semi-circular fold of skin that overlaps the nail plate on either side is called the nail wall. In order to allow the nail to move when it grows there is a nail groove on each side of the nail plate. Beneath the skin at the base of the nail there is a deep fold of skin called the nail mantle, in

Your efforts so far will appear totally worthless if you neglect your fingernails. Ragged, bitten and broken nails look scruffy and untidy so it is well worthwhile taking care of them. Picture courtesy of Perfect Colour by Cutex.

which the nail root is found. The hyponychium is the skin located directly below the nail's free edge. The skin that surrounds the entire nail is the perionychium, and, most important is the matrix, or the inner part of the nail, which affects the nail's shape, size and growth. This contains all the blood vessels and nerve cells it needs to help the nail grow, and it is here that the protein keratin grows and hardens. If the matrix is injured the growth and shape of the nail can be distorted.

Nail problems

Nails grow continuously at the rate of one millimetre per day, and they grow faster in summer than winter. If a nail is lost or removed it will take about three months to restore – three times that amount if it is a toenail. Your general physical and emotional state is also reflected in the state of your nails and, if you are suffering from illness or nervous tension, nail growth is affected. Obviously there are some nail conditions that should be referred to a doctor, but many of the common injuries to which we submit our nails can be avoided. It takes only a little time and effort, with careful consideration and regular manicures, to make the most of these sadly neglected, and underrated, beauty assets.

Nail biting is probably our fingernail's worst enemy, but it is a nervous habit that can be stopped with a little effort and determination. Otherwise you may risk not just badly deformed nails but disease from the bacteria on the nails or infection of the cuticle from the bacteria in your mouth. Willpower is your greatest ally, but you can try applying distasteful nail enamels and chemicals to help you break the habit, and start pampering your nails on a regular basis to help them look neat and tidy.

If your nail appears to lose its sheen and the plate decreases in size and seems to separate from the nail bed you are suffering from onychatrophia, or atrophy of the nails. This can be caused by injury to the matrix or internal disease. Treat your nail with a fine emery board – never use a metal file – and avoid subjecting your nails to highly alkaline soap or detergents. Small tears or nail splits which bleed and become painfully raw are hangnails. This is a fairly common complaint and can be caused by dryness or injury, perhaps as a result of tearing or improper filing. If only a small area of skin is affected, soak it in an antiseptic solution and you will find that the skin will rebuild fairly quickly. If a large area is involved, then seek the advice of your doctor.

White spots on the nail are nothing to worry about. They can be hereditary or the result of injury, but they will grow out as the nail grows. Split, brittle nails are sometimes caused by injury to the nail or by strong solvents, such as some nail enamels and nail-polish removers. If this is your problem, then consult a beautician for a hot-oil manicure to really condition your nails or alternatively seek help and advice from your doctor.

As you can see, most common nail complaints, such as fragile, split and brittle nails, can be alleviated and eventually conquered with regular care and attention. Protect your nails by wearing rubber gloves when they are likely to come into contact with daily cleaning agents like washing-up liquid and scouring powder. Feed them with creams on a daily basis to help make them more supple, and protect them with special enamel strengtheners. Also keep them a moderate length, as there will then be less chance of them breaking, and they will be easier to keep clean and in good condition. Personally, I really do think that shorter, neat nails look nicer than long talons.

Manicure

Treat yourself to a manicure, if not a professional one then a home one, once a week. This will enable you to detect anything that may be wrong with your nails before it gets out of hand – also it's another way of making you sit down and relax for 10 minutes, which can't be a bad thing. The actual process of the manicure frees the cuticle and nail wall from the nail plate, avoiding the risk of hangnails, and the outline of the nail will be kept smooth and infection thus prevented.

Before you sit down to do your manicure gather all your necessary tools around you. You'll need cotton wool, nail-varnish remover, cuticle cream, cuticle remover, a finger bowl, towel, scissors, emery boards, cuticle scissors, orange sticks, a metal pusher, base coat, nail enamel and top coat, buffer and hand cream. First remove any traces of nail enamel, and this includes nail strengthener which may have peeled or chipped off, with decisive movements. A cotton-wool pad soaked in remover may have to be applied to the nail for a few seconds to thoroughly remove varnish from a heavily painted nail. Then take an orange stick, soaked in remover, and clean up the cuticles and edges to make sure all traces of polish are removed. Think about your nail shape. There are four basic nail shapes – round, oval, pointed and square. Use a coarse emery board and shape the nail from one side towards the centre, never with the back and forth sawing technique I see most people using. You can perform no better hatchet job on your nail, as this action will cause it to split and crack. Tilt the board slightly so that it touches the bottom side of the nail's free edge, and work with smooth, quick, short strokes. Use the fine side of the emery board to lightly file the edge of the nail downwards and complete the shape.

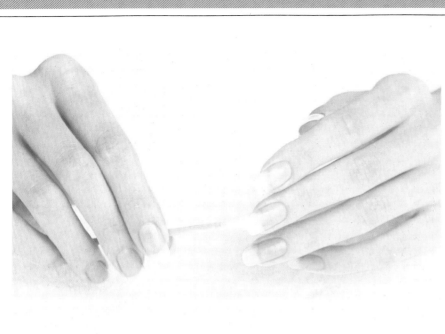

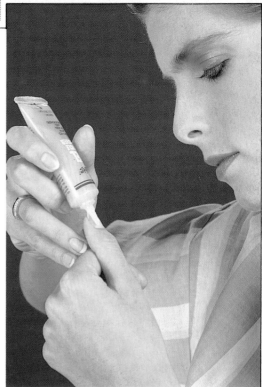

Above: In the same way that your face has to be spotlessly clean before you apply make-up, so do your nails. *Above right:* Eliminating overgrown cuticles is an essential part of any manicure. This cuticle remover gel can be dispensed from the tube. Pictures courtesy of Sally Hansen. *Main picture, right:* Nail enamel should be applied in three definite strokes. Picture courtesy of Perfect Colour by Cutex.

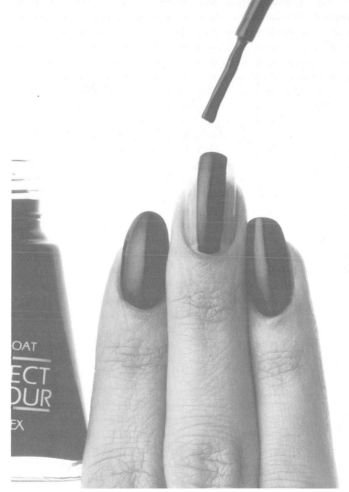

Once both hands are filed, dip them in warm, soapy water to enable the cuticle to soften. With a cotton-tipped orange stick, apply cuticle remover to each free edge and cuticle and gently push the cuticle back to the fold of the skin. Check that the nails are clean underneath, and if necessary, clean them with a cotton-tipped orange stick. Now get rid of any excess cuticle remover with a towel. Next apply a little cuticle cream to each nail, working it into the nail plate and surrounding tissue. This strengthens these areas and discourages the appearance of hangnails. Remove any ragged cuticles with a special cuticle nipper. Now apply hand lotion and massage it well into your hands, even up to the elbows if you feel like it.

If required, nail strengthener should be applied at this stage.

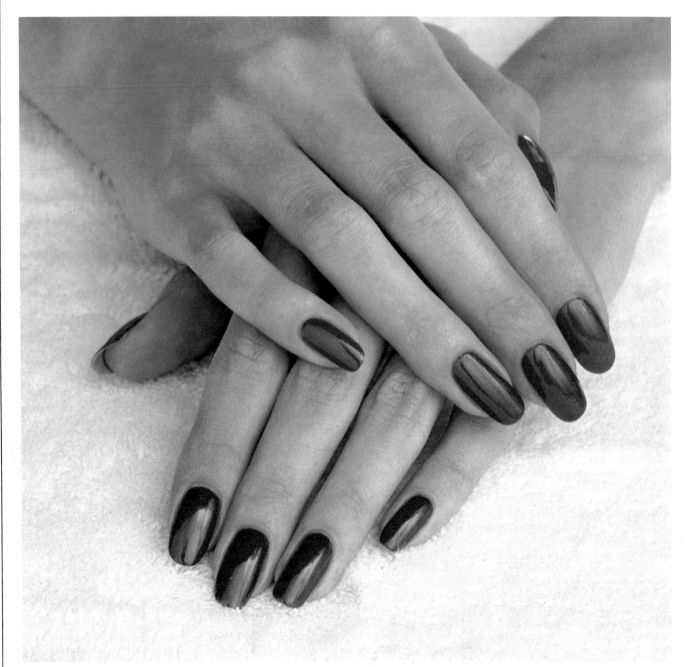

Once you've achieved a perfectly polished set of nails, don't allow them to get chipped. Try preserving them with a nightly application of cuticle cream. Picture courtesy of Sally Hansen.

Work with light, fast strokes to prevent smudging and ensure an even coverage, just as you would apply coloured nail enamel. If you are wearing a cream nail varnish you'll probably need a top coat to add lustre, although this is usually unnecessary for pearly enamels. Unless you have all day to allow them to dry, keep the varnish down to four coats or less – base, two coloured coats and a top coat if required. Any enamel which touches the nail wall during application should be removed before you go any further since, once it sets, it will be impossible to remove it cleanly and without smudging. Always apply enamel in three strokes, the first in the centre from the base of the nail to the tip, and then one on each side. Boost your manicure with a nightly application of cuticle cream massaged all over, including the nail enamel, to the folds of the skin. Needless to say, if you ever allowed yourself to be seen in public with chipped nail varnish, you might as well not have bothered in the first place! If you haven't got time to re-apply or patch up, remove the enamel altogether. Clean, well-shaped fingernails look far more presentable than painted, cracked ones.

False nails

If you are an incurable nail nibbler or feel you lack the patience to manicure your own nails, don't despair — all is not lost. Artificial nails provide an ideal temporary glamour coverage but aren't terribly durable. The best answer is nail extensions, which provide a fairly long-lasting way of disguising broken nails or of helping to grow out bitten ones without looking too artificial. However, it has to be stressed that nail extensions should only be applied by a beautician or in a salon specializing in the work, as the process involves dealing with substances which could be harmful to the nail if not applied professionally. Nail extensions can be used to lengthen natural nails, either a whole set or one at a time, if all you want to do is repair a damaged nail until it grows to match the others. Extensions stay in place until the nail has grown sufficiently for the extension to be unnecessary.

Nail extensions are basically the modern answer to artificial nails. They rely on a tough, fast-acting glue to bond the plastic nail shape to the natural nail. One stage further than this are the semi-permanent nail additions, where compounds are applied to cover the nails entirely and extend their natural length. Abrasive drills are used to shape these compounds. This treatment requires regular in-filling as the nail grows, so that the nail addition is kept looking as natural as possible. This is more of a grooming service than a repair one, since it takes longer to perform, but the results are much more long lasting and often worth the effort.

Can you begin to imagine how unfinished these ladies would look without varnish on their nails? Four coats should be sufficient: a base coat, two coloured coats and a top coat. Any enamel which touches the nail wall during application should be removed immediately as, once its set, it won't come off easily and smudges of colour outside of the nail will look messy. Nail varnishes vary tremendously in price but these, from Dior, seem to last very well.

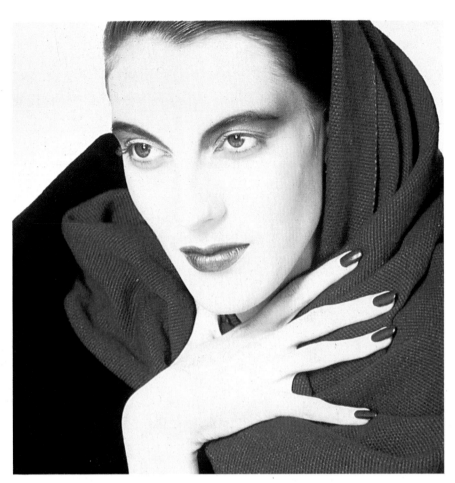

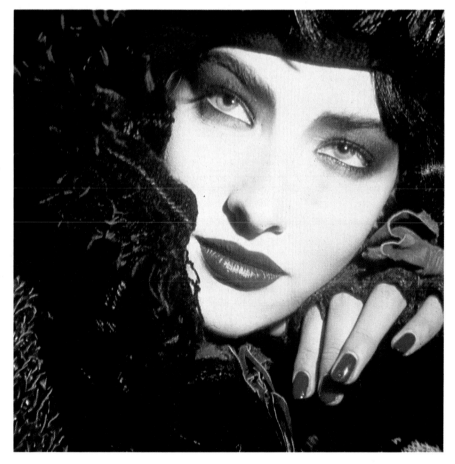

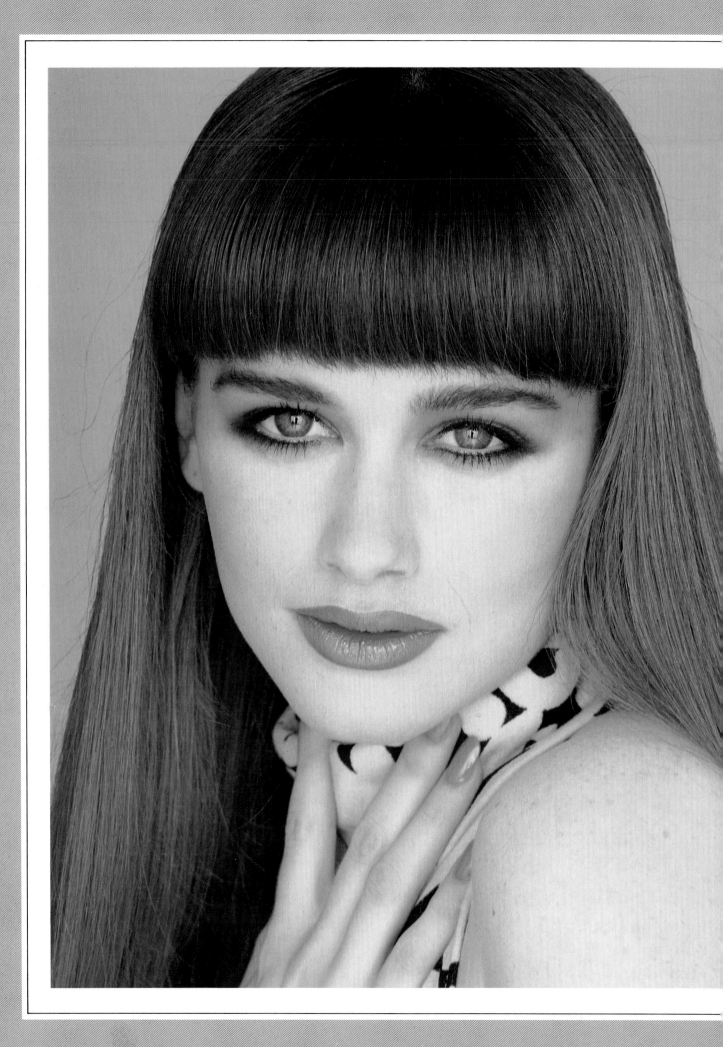

Finishing touches

I cannot end this book without a few words on the finer points of appearance, the lack of which very often let a person down. Have you ever heard that phrase 'She's a funny girl, she looks absolutely dreadful, but she's really ever so nice'? For me it's all too familiar, but I always feel it's a crying shame when a person's personality isn't reflected in the way they look. It is one of life's sad facts that we are each of us judged every day by appearances. A women is actually quite lucky, as she has so many opportunities to build up her personality by creating her total image to suit it. Make-up is just one, albeit very important, aspect but there are others of equal importance.

Foot care

Let's start from the feet and work upwards. I'm not about to give a lecture on how badly we neglect our feet, but they are important, for comfort as much as for anything else, and we should look after them. The best way to treat them is to invest in good, comfortable, well-fitting shoes; pamper them, and don't be a martyr to fashion. If you've never had a pedicure then you've been missing

You must never forget your crowning glory which can make, or break, your total look. Work at getting your hair into peak condition as hard as you will now be working at getting your skin clear and radiant. Picture courtesy of Perfect Colour by Cutex.

out. Nothing relaxed me more when I was expecting my baby than a weekly pedicure, and I'm someone who, until the age of 20, couldn't bear to have her toes touched! Don't misunderstand the purpose of a pedicure. Complaints like ingrowing toenails, corns and callouses should all be referred to a chiropodist. A pedicure is simply a manicure of the feet; it will perk and pretty them up, but it can't perform miracles. If you are going to do it yourself at home, and it really is a cheap treat, you'll need clean towels, a large foot bowl, foot powder, nail clippers, soap or antiseptic solution, a hard-skin remover, a soothing, skin-softening lotion, cuticle remover, orange sticks, and, if you decide to use it, nail enamel. I'm not a great lover of nail varnish, but I think that in the summer, nothing does more for brown feet in open-toed sandals than a light covering of apricot or pink nail enamel on the toes.

First allow your feet to soak in the bowl, filled with warm water and a soapy, disinfectant solution. Work on one foot at a time. Dry the first thoroughly, remove any nail enamel and trim the nails by cutting them straight across, leaving only a gentle curve at the sides to prevent ingrowing toenails. File the nails with a metal file to remove any rough edges. Remove any adhering cuticle skin in the same way you would with your fingernails, with cuticle remover and an orange stick. Now remove any hard skin on the heels and toe

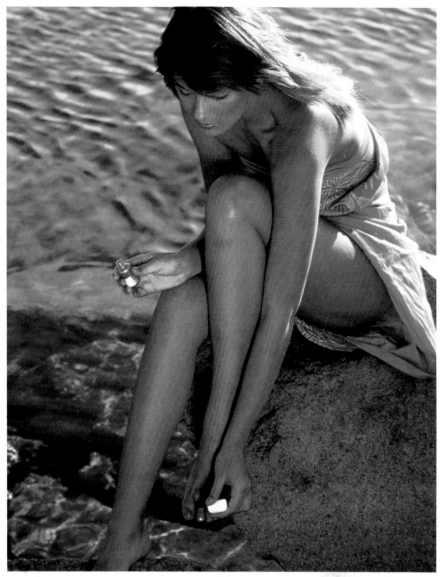

Total beauty is about looking good from top to bottom, so please don't forget those feet, they do take an awful lot of wear and tear. Pamper them occasionally by giving them a pedicure to make them feel wanted! Picture courtesy of Dior.

Style

No woman can dictate to another the way she should dress. Some people have an innate sense of style, while others have none and need all the guidance they can get. But it can only be guidance, for every woman should be able to adapt what she buys to suit herself. If you wear nothing but Dior from head to toe you will look like a Dior mannequin, and not an ounce of your own personality will be reflected.

For someone who tries hard but doesn't always quite get it right, and who is constantly making comparisons with French and Italian women who somehow always manage to make their clothes work for them, here are a few tips learnt the hard way. Never think cheap; the saving of a few pounds is a false economy. Cheap clothes look cheap, they crumple and crease easily and they don't travel well. Don't fall foul of fashion; use it as a guideline to dress up and enhance what you already have rather than as a dictate. Moderately priced or more expensive clothes really do keep their fashion appeal and style for much longer than their cheaper counterparts. Never buy on the spur-of-the-moment or just for the sake of it. Always go home and think about if first. That shirt you loved so much in the shop might fade into oblivion when placed with the six you already have in the wardrobe, or it might not go with any of your existing clothes, so that you will have to rush out and buy something else to wear with it! If your pocket ever allows you, invest in one or two good outfits that you'll always be able to rely on. Mine are a brown suede trouser suit and a black cocktail dress. The accessories change but they never do; they travel everywhere with me and are absolutely invaluable.

Good accessories are the key to class. They make the difference between an outfit which looks just

pad areas and place the foot back in the bowl while you do exactly the same thing to the other foot. Now take both feet out of the bowl and dry them thoroughly. Apply your soothing lotion in firm movements from the base of the toes towards the ankles. To apply the nail enamel, put rolled-up pieces of cotton wool between the toes of the first foot. Apply a base coat and then the enamel in the same way you would apply it to fingernails, with three firm, decisive strokes, one down the centre and then one on each side. Make sure the nails are dry before you remove the cotton wool.

One aspect of foot care that many of us forget is to keep our footwear clean and in good condition. Always have your shoes repaired before the damage is too great, and always wipe them over with a cloth or shoe brush every day before you go out. A good way of avoiding scuffing around the heels of shoes, which can make the most expensive pair look tatty, and is sometimes impossible to rectify, is to keep an old pair of flatties in the car for driving in and use them whenever you drive, even if it's just to go down the road to get the shopping. It will save you a fortune in shoe repairs!

okay and one which looks wonderful. Chunky earrings, a multi-coloured wrap, a good leather belt and tights in every colour all help to give an outfit that certain something. Always think about where you are going before you dress for the day. If you're going to be sitting down a lot or travelling make sure your attire doesn't crease easily. Silk is disastrous; only wear it if you know your are going to be on your feet for eight hours! There is no excuse for laddered or darned tights. Always pack a new pair, matching your outfit, in your handbag.

Finishing touches

Always take a long, last lingering look in the mirror before you go out for the day. How do your clothes look and feel? It may be great to be wearing a pair of trousers a size smaller than your usual, but if they make your bottom appear to bulge it won't be compliments you are paid by passers-by. Make sure your underwear is right for your clothes; knicker lines look terrible.

The absolute crowning glory of any woman's looks is her hair. The right hairstyle can do so much to boost a woman's confidence and, since it is the one part of her 'wardrobe' she can't, very easily, take off, it is essential to get it right. Find a good hairdresser who really cares about you and invest in regular trims and conditioning treatments. And if you are really interested read my book *The Hamlyn Basic Guide to Hair Care and Styling.*

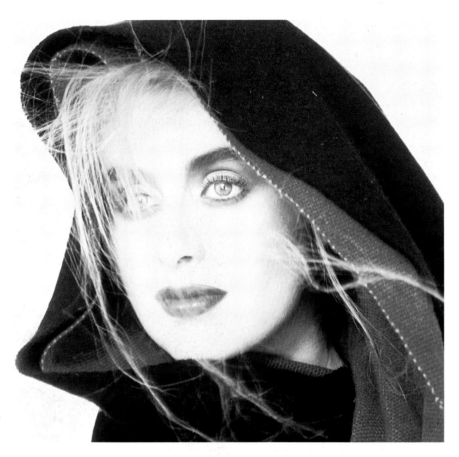

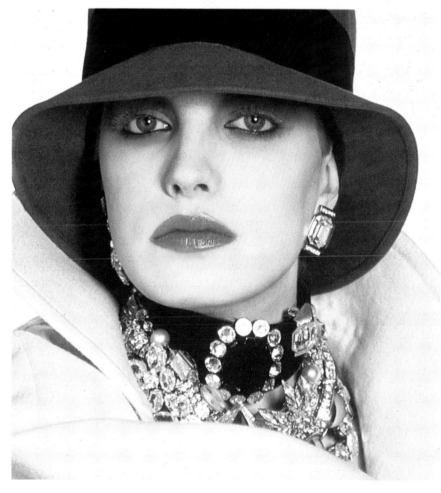

For a completely well-groomed look, don't forget to add accessories to your appearance. These little extras can make the world of difference to an outfit, and even make an inexpensive one look like a designer label. The romantic mood above is accentuated with the use of a cape while below, a look of sleek sophistication is made complete with the use of a hat. Pictures courtesy of Dior.

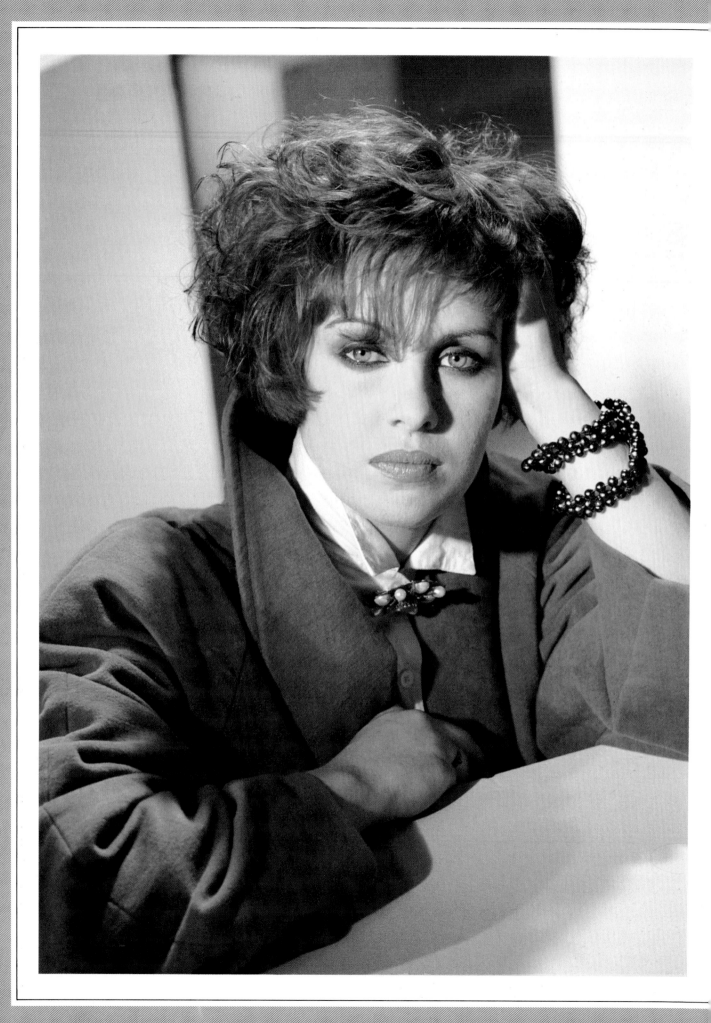

Index

The epitome of the total look. Hair, clothes, make-up and jewellery are all colour co-ordinated and well matched. Everything looks as if it has been thought about, and it has. And with a little application it doesn't take that much forethought. Picture courtesy of Alan International.

Acknowledgments

The author wishes to thank the following people and organizations who have especially helped with the preparation of this book: Clinique, Katherine Corbett, Christian Dior, Max Factor and Liz Michael.